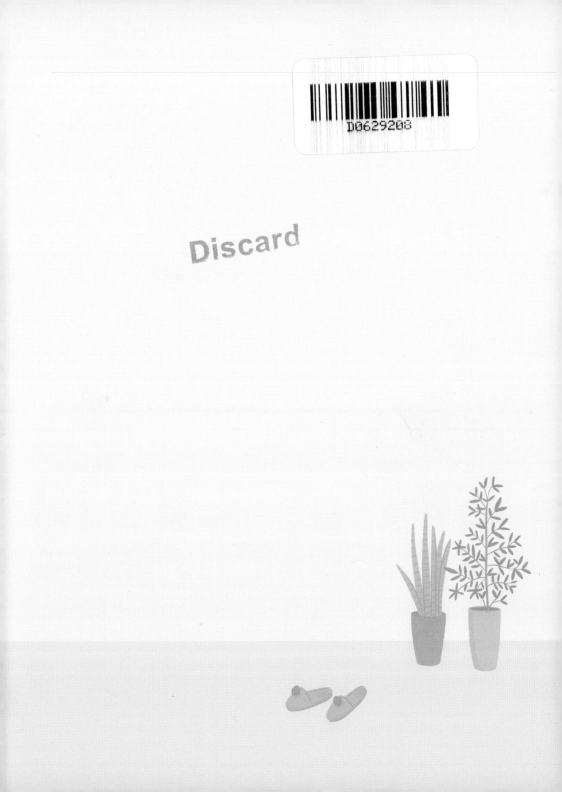

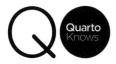

Brimming with creative inspiration, how-to projects and useful information to enrich your everyday life, Quarto Knows is a favourite destination for those pursuing their interests and passions. Visit our site and dig deeper with our books into your area of interest: Quarto Creates, Quarto Cooks, Quarto Homes, Quarto Lives, Quarto Drives, Quarto Explores, Quarto Gifts, or Quarto Kids.

First published in 2019 by White Lion Publishing, an imprint of The Quarto Group. The Old Brewery, 6 Blundell Street London, N7 9BH, United Kingdom T (0)20 7700 6700 www.QuartoKnows.com

A catalogue record for this book is available from the British Library.

ISBN 978 1 78131 916 1
Ebook ISBN 978 1 78131 917 8

10 9 8 7 6 5 4 3 2 1

Design by Isabel Eeles
Illustrations by Amelia Flower

Printed in China

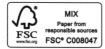

THE SERENITY PASSPORT

A world tour of peaceful
living in 30 words

MEGAN C HAYES PhD

Illustrated by
AMELIA FLOWER

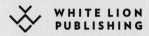
WHITE LION
PUBLISHING

Contents

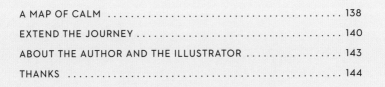

Serenity
Around
the
World

In a frantic world, finding pockets of serenity can be tricky. We feel there is always somewhere else to be, someone else to link up with in the digital world, some other goal to achieve... Yet most of us recognise the importance of taking time to relax and 'unplug', even if we do not always practise what we preach.

Interestingly, no matter in what corner of the globe we find ourselves, in all kinds of climates, across all languages and dialects, we humans are adept at finding clever ways to keep calm. Over time, this has manifested into a treasure trove of distinct terms, concepts and practices that our many cultures prize and revere; from ancient philosophical ideas to contemporary ways of relaxing.

Some of these words and practices are about finding a peaceful sense of wellbeing collectively, while others are about retreating and finding serenity in moments of quiet solitude. At their heart, all of these concepts reflect how, alone and together, we treasure tranquillity.

What we can learn from 'untranslatable' words & practices

Why search out - with the appropriate cultural sensitivity - the wisdom of languages beyond our own for ways of living calmer lives? First and foremost is that this helps us question our status quo. Despite our best efforts, all cultures and communities are at risk of becoming blinkered to our own way of doing things. Secondly, when it comes to calm, in seeking a wider range of wisdom we can discover answers to questions we have been unable to solve. Finally, we might just feel more connected to our global compatriots.

Ironically, in our digitally connected world, it is in many ways easier than ever to feel disconnected. The wisdom of the ages – and of each other – can be all too easily lost in a flurry of online distractions; from instantly accessible box sets, to seeking 'likes' on social media, to addictive apps.

Yet when we stop to really listen to the world around us, we uncover long-held approaches to even our most contemporary of problems, whether that is world-weariness, anxiety, loneliness or isolation from one another. We also discover how differing cultures, near and far, find quirky new approaches to these age-old challenges all the time.

In seeking to share these answers and ideas – from the past and present, and across cultures and continents – we realise that people might change, but the roots of our problems often do not (such as how to keep our cool in a sometimes arduous and uncertain world). By deciphering these 'untranslatable' ways of living peaceful lives, we can find new and perhaps far more profound ways to feel allied with one another and become calmer still as a result.

How these words were chosen

This book has been arranged in five chapters to offer a sense of the very different ways in which we can both understand and practise serenity in our lives. They are not prescriptive and, naturally, many concepts have not made it into these pages. This is in the hope of achieving as broad and surprising a representation as possible. This book, of course, is not an effort to compile an exhaustive account of how calm and serenity manifest around our world, but rather offers an initial glimpse at the marvellous variety of these expressions.

A celebration of serenity

Above all, this book is a celebration. These varied and distinct colourings of calm reflect the many ways in which, with astonishing tenacity, human beings find peaceful ways to live. Let us be in awe of the steadfastness of the human spirit in choosing serenity, again and again, in our efforts to live well.

A NOTE FROM THE AUTHOR

Writing a book that draws upon so many divergent languages and traditions is not without its pitfalls. While I have made every effort to portray these terms and practices accurately, their 'untranslatable' nature has made this a richly complex and delicate task. It has been my great privilege to gather and compile this collection as precisely and sensitively as possible, and I only hope that the generous reader will excuse me any accidental imprecisions.

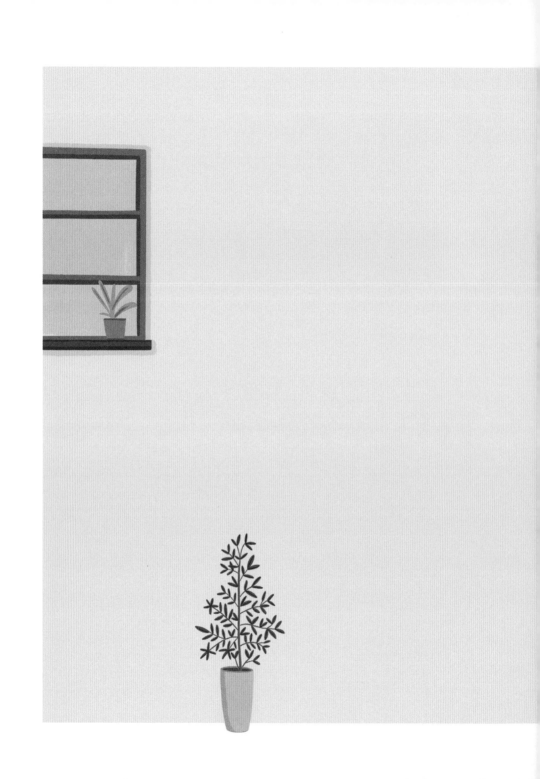

CHAPTER ONE

Focus & Awareness

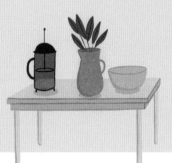

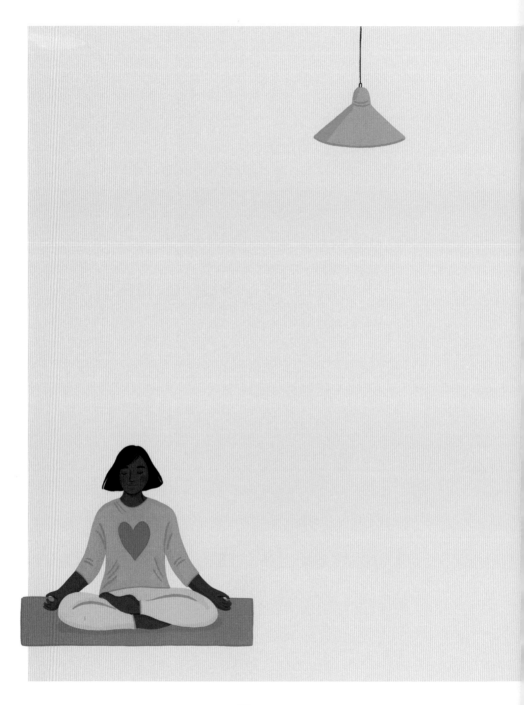

With an ever more enticing range of technological tools at our disposal, life in the developed world comes with a side dish of constant distraction. We check our email as soon as we wake up, get social media updates while we work and keep our phones bleeping away beside our beds at night. Simply put: in the modern age we find ourselves on call for the wider world twenty-four hours a day, every day. This is a sure-fire recipe for anxiety and, as such, many of us now look for ways that we can consciously slow down, catch our breath and unplug from the incessant buzz of the Internet.

While this may seem like a very modern dilemma, it turns out that all over the world humans have been trying to keep our cool and stay focussed for centuries (it is only the distractions that change). From the philosophy of ancient China and the intricate belief system of Buddhism to cultures as distinctive as those of Bulgaria or Hawaii – all around the planet we have cultivated clever and treasured techniques to help us be more mindful.

These various practices remind us to stay in the moment and make sure we regularly reflect upon what is important to us. We can use these humble techniques and preferred pastimes to help us avoid becoming distracted by the onslaught of duties and dilemmas we all face, and to keep our minds calmly and resolutely focussed on our highest values. These values might include caring for the people we love, looking out for our wider communities, adhering to our ethical principles or just keeping our commitment to enjoy the moment. Let us take a whirlwind tour of how, in some very distinctive corners of our world, we opt to focus our attention and stay serene.

SHU (恕)

(Pinyin): shù | noun | Traditional Chinese
1. the Confucian virtue of compassion and concern for others

Many of us consider those we love to be at the centre of our lives, but if we stop to think about it we may find we actually spend very little time in the average day devoted to conscious reflection upon these cherished others. More than this, human beings often rely on the kindness of complete strangers; an idea reflected through folklore and fairy tales since time immemorial. Yet how much is this intertwinement with others reflected in the flurry of our daily activities? Perhaps not much at all.

Across cultures, languages, nations and religions we find variants of something that we in the West like to call The Golden Rule. This directive poses that in living our lives justly we should strive to treat others how we ourselves wish to be treated. This idea is a pretty useful one because, well, it renders everyone a winner. It is this spirit that is precisely captured in the traditional Chinese concept of *shu* (恕), which stems from Confucian philosophy and encapsulates concern and care for others. In modern Chinese usage, this word can also mean to forgive, to show mercy to or to accommodate others.

What is perhaps most fascinating about the concept of *shu* is that when we focus our minds on others in this way it is not only good for others, it is good for us too. In fact, it is a strong motivation for humans to be connected to one another and to belong – some psychologists would say it is our primary motivation. It therefore does wonders for our wellbeing to cultivate a sense of belonging. Yet in the hustle and bustle of the average week, as we hurry from commitment to commitment, it is all too easy to forget to make the space to focus on others, which may leave us feeling fraught and cut off. Make some time this week to reflect with care upon someone other than you – someone close, or someone who may as yet be a stranger – and let the desire to belong that is captured by *shu* guide your way of living.

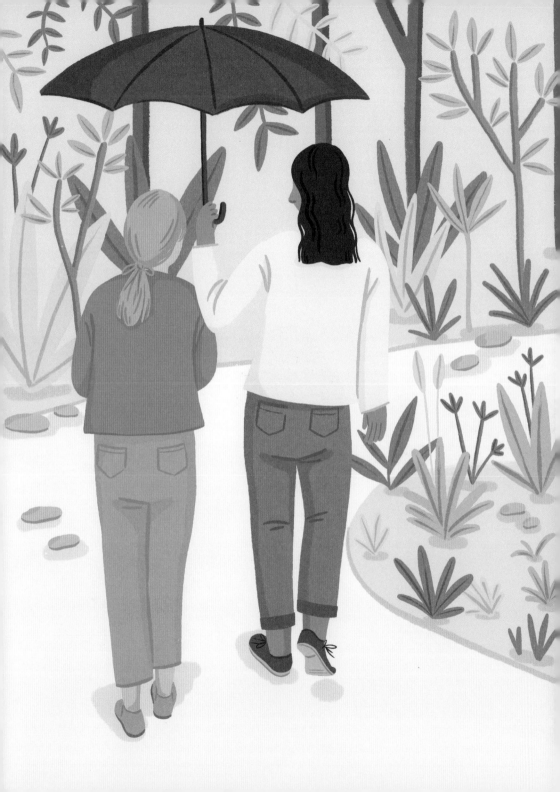

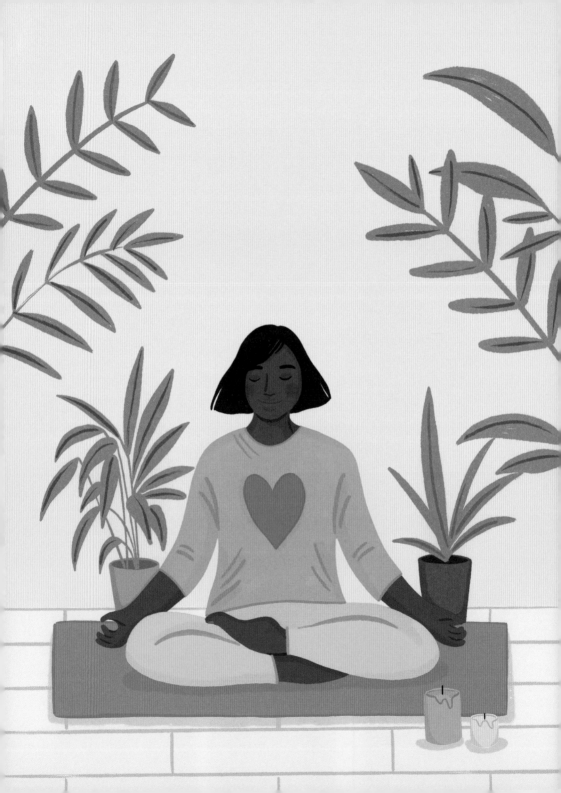

TRY THIS...

Loving-Kindness Meditation

Have a go at this helpful practice that puts the beautiful virtue of shu into action for a calmer and more consciously caring day. There are many ways to meditate. You might focus on your breathing; try any number of calming visualisations; or conduct a 'body scan' whereby you gradually notice and release tension in your body. Yet one meditation practice that makes a point of focusing compassionately on others (in the spirit of *shu*) is Loving-Kindness Meditation. There are variations on how you can go about this practice, but the essential aim is that you extend compassion to others, either real or imagined, along with sincere wishes of wellbeing.

A typical meditation of this kind involves a step-by-step process:

1. Begin by sitting quietly with closed eyes and simply focus upon your commitment to your own wellbeing and feelings of deep compassion for yourself, exactly as you are in this moment.

2. Following some minutes of this, carry these feelings into thinking about someone you know and love, beginning to extend similar feelings of care and well wishes to them.

3. Finally, extend these same considerate feelings to the wider world, reflecting upon your sense of deep compassion and kindness towards all beings.

For the true aficionados of the Loving-Kindness approach to meditation, there is also the option to include an extra step of extending feelings of compassion to somebody with whom you may be experiencing a troublesome or difficult relationship; perhaps even someone you consider a rival or enemy. With trial and error, extending well wishes to these otherwise bothersome individuals can be a useful way of remaining unruffled in the face of challenging work or family relationships – and is something to aim for as you build this compassionate, calming habit into your life.

This practice not only feels good, it has tangible benefits. One group of psychologists at Stanford University found that even a brief Loving-Kindness meditation offered a clear boost to the sense of social connectedness in those involved in the study, and even increased their feelings of positivity and compassion towards complete strangers. Certainly, then, this looks like one surefire way to put the essence of *shu* to good use in your day-to-day life.

SATI

sʌˈtiː | noun | Pāli
1. memory; recognition   2. mindfulness

Mindfulness has become a familiar concept around the world, yet we do not often hear of its origins, namely in the word *sati* found in the Pāli Canon – the sacred writings of the Theravada Buddhist tradition. While *sati* principally refers to the type of meditational awareness that has been translated into English as 'mindfulness', it is a term that is broad in scope and has many other connotations. Aside from referring to attentiveness, *sati* can refer to a kind of remembering, or what one Pāli scholar calls non-forgetfulness.

   This idea – that being mindful is about being non-forgetful – is a vital one if we wish to grasp the ancient concept of *sati*. Think about it: how much of your life is spent in an autopilot state of forgetfulness? For example when you are handed a train or bus ticket and almost instantly lose it because you hide it away somewhere absent-mindedly. To be truly mindful is, in some ways, to remember to notice each moment as it occurs.

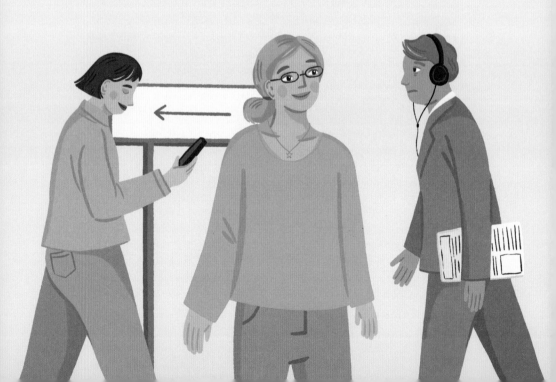

Sati is a wakeful state in which we are alert to the information being received by our five senses, without judgement or assessment, just simply being in the experience. In this state, we are able to act as an observer and interpreter of this data; noticing how such input translates into thoughts and feelings. By being mindfully observant in this way, the idea is that we can stand apart from our constantly whirring thoughts – a truly calming state if we can achieve it.

Yet, isolating the idea of *sati* from the rich tradition of Buddhist teachings means, inevitably, many of its nuances are lost. Though the full context is too intricate to be captured here, an important element to note is that one of the ultimate teachings of Buddhism is to do away with the idea of an *observer*, or self, altogether, and to become aware of our own impermanence. Whether your voyage into mindfulness will take you this far is for you to decide, but one thing is for sure: a little more non-forgetfulness, or *sati*, could mean a little less stress.

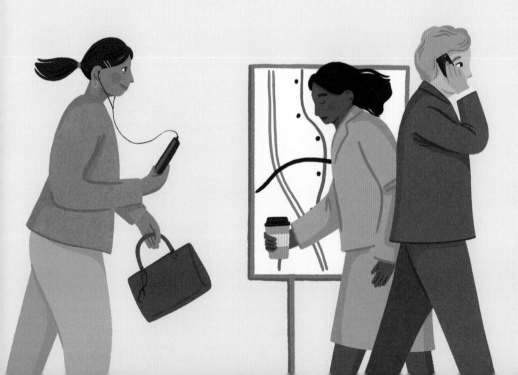

TRY THIS...

Three Ways to a More Mindful Day

We do not necessarily have to become masters of meditation to benefit from mindfulness. To make *sati* a practice in your own life, here are three straightforward ways to begin being more mindful daily.

Take a more mindful shower

One of the best ways to establish a new habit is to connect it with something we are already doing regularly. We do not normally have to convince ourselves to brush our teeth or take a shower – these are non-negotiable and intrinsic parts of our day. So why not make these activities more mindful and strive to become completely focussed on the activity? In your daily shower, practise *sati* or non-forgetfulness, observing the different kinds of input your senses are receiving. How does the hot water feel? How does it sound against the shower tray? What does your soap or shampoo smell like? What is it like to see through the steam? Starting out with this simple activity will help you to carry this alert awareness into the rest of your day.

Sit more mindfully

One of the places we are least likely to be in a state of *sati* is when sitting at our desks or around the table of a staff meeting. Yet even here we can benefit from mindfulness. Next time you notice yourself stressed and tense in a chair, take a few slow breaths and direct your attention to your feet as you place them firmly to the floor. How do they feel? Notice how they press into the ground. Wiggle your toes and keep your awareness there for a moment. Spend a few minutes this way, gently drawing your attention back to your feet whenever it wanders. This is an easy mindful exercise to help you gently centre yourself in times of stress.

Do some mindful journal writing

The practice of *sati* is about noticing life as it happens, and one of the easiest ways to cultivate this kind of wakeful awareness is to write things down. As you go about your day, make a point of noticing unusual, beautiful or surprising things that you see. It might be the evening light through the trees, traffic lights reflected in a puddle, or an interesting looking person on the train – whatever captures your attention. Then, in the evening, take a few moments to note these things in a journal, contemplating why they intrigued you. The idea of this practice is that noticing what is going on around us will then become a habit, and we will begin to mindfully perceive the poetic beauty of even the most seemingly mundane of days.

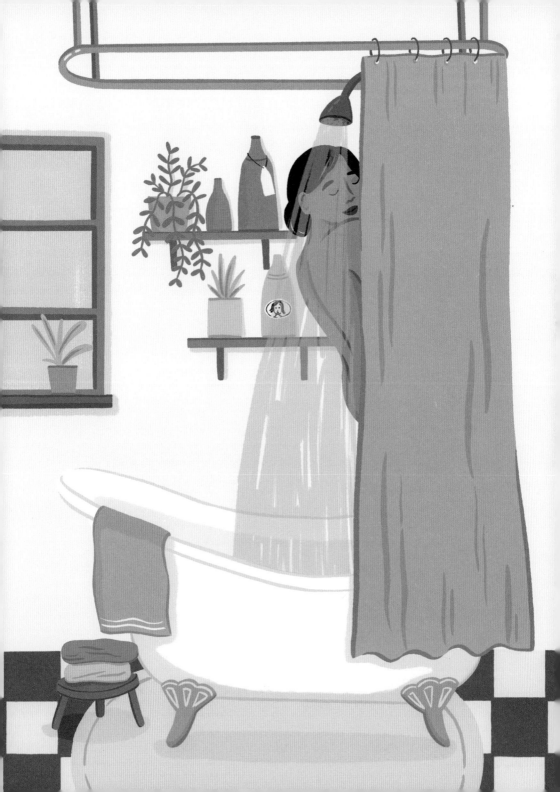

IT'S IN OUR NATURE...
TAKE A DIGITAL DETOX AND SEEK
CALM IN THE OUTSIDE WORLD

If our aim is to find focus in today's modern world, sadly the odds are not often in our favour. In any given home or workspace we are bombarded with technological stimulus. Our phones are never more than an arm's length away, our computers and televisions flash on at the touch of a button and transport us to the never-ending rabbit hole of the digital realm, and now even our fridges and appliances are becoming 'smart'. While we can certainly establish practices that help us drown out this digital buzz, sometimes the only thing for it is to step outdoors for a full digital detox.

In many languages we find terms, both fun and philosophical, promoting the peaceful joy of being in nature. In woodlands and up mountains, in fields, glens and valleys, on cool winter days or bright hot summer ones – there are perhaps as many ways to find peace and tranquility in nature as there are coastlines to sit beside or mountain paths to traverse. In fact, we find joyful calm in the outside world in all weathers (in Icelandic, *hoppípolla* is a verb for jumping in puddles).

One portion of the natural world, however, that appears to have a particularly profound influence upon our sense of calm – and often plays a big part in our appreciation of the calming influence of the great outdoors – is the humble tree. The Russians have a noun for the 'falling leaves' from trees – *listopad* (листопад) – bringing to mind the gentle passing of time that seasonal forests so poetically evoke. Time in the woods is relaxing because our senses are gently stirred by such sounds, and also by that special kind of light found only beneath canopies of boughs and branches.

The Japanese love trees, too, and have both *komorebi* (木漏れ日), a term to describe the beauty of sunlight filtering through leaves; and *shinrin-yoku* (森林浴) or 'forest-bathing' – like sunbathing but soaking up the dappled and tranquil forest instead of rays.

AYLIAK (АЙЛЯК)

aɪlaɪk | noun | Bulgarian
1. Bulgarian: the art of living slowly and without worries

Despite our best efforts to stay focussed and calm, few of us are immune to worry. Worrying can at times feel like an inherent part of modern existence, so much so that we may not notice we are even doing it. Our fast-paced lifestyles seem to dictate this way of being; haste and anxiety masquerade as perfectly natural, necessary responses to a hectic schedule. Yet much of this comes down, not to necessity, but to our priorities – and not all nations, cities or cultures prioritise in the same way.

Take the Bulgarian people and their concept of *Ayliak* (Айляк), which originates from the Turkish word for 'idle'. In Bulgarian, however, this word implies a specific 'culture of slowness' that cannot be characterised as simple idleness. *Ayliak* evokes that one's main concern is a lifestyle of calm living, free from worry and stress.

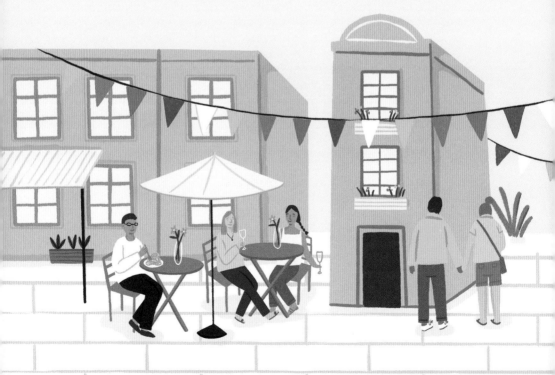

It is said that this word is particularly unique to (and typical of) the people of Plovdiv, Bulgaria's second-biggest city. We might associate big cities with fast-paced lifestyles, but Plovdiv is a place where a serene existence is a local pastime. The citizens of Plovdiv are famous in Bulgaria for living with the spirit of *Ayliak*: prioritising the unhurried and harmonious over the hectic and frenetic. In particular, they are known for expressing this philosophy through their slow-paced strolls around the city.

So proud are the citizens of Plovdiv about this cultural quirk that they have developed not one but two festivals in honour of the term: the *Ayliak* (I LIKE) festival and The Slow City Fest. For many of us, 'Slow City' might seem like a contradiction in terms. For Plovdivians, it is a part of who they are: a shared commitment to forgo busyness for relaxed enjoyment of life, one unhurried moment at a time.

Wherever you find yourself in the world – big city, small town or otherwise – the people of Plovdiv show that sometimes it is our priorities and not the place in which we find ourselves that define how we focus our minds.

FLOW

flǝʊ | noun | English
1. (psychology) a state of energised focus and awareness
in an activity; being immersed or 'in the zone'

Our world's many philosophical traditions have reflected upon the human mind for millennia, including how we choose to direct our awareness. Yet it is only since the mid-1800s that this preoccupation has been formalised into a scientific discipline: the study of psychology. Out of this discipline have come innumerable new ways to understand the mind and gain a 'big picture' overview of how individuals and communities across the globe both survive and thrive. One particularly fascinating concept to emerge from this tradition is the idea of *flow*.

Flow is an English term coined by Hungarian-American psychologist Mihaly Csikszentmihalyi after he studied groups of highly motivated people passionate about various recreational activities – from musical composition, to rock climbing, to ballet dancing. These groups described how such experiences fully engaged their minds, carrying them along almost like a current of water. Thus *flow* gives a name to the state of intense and pleasurable focus, where our awareness of time, place, personal problems – and even of our very selves – is temporarily suspended in a way that is both calming and fulfilling.

What is helpfully captured by this term is something long-known and practised in many far flung corners of our world, particularly in Eastern traditions such as Buddhism: the idea that the quality of our attention matters, and that we can exercise ways of focussing that are conducive to greater wellbeing. The opposite of *flow* experience, then, might be the Buddhist notion of the 'monkey mind', where our thoughts jump inconsistently and feverishly from one thing to another, and we struggle to give our attention to the moment. This idea highlights how our attention is a *resource* at our disposal – something we can actively use to our advantage to bring us joy, calm and greater wellbeing.

Flow – like focus – can arise in many different ways depending upon the person, from walking, to reading a good book or getting lost in a lively conversation. Its defining features are simply that we forget where, and even who, we are for a little while: a kind of sublime narrowing of our attention to the simple moment-to-moment unfolding of our experience, in a way that is deeply rewarding.

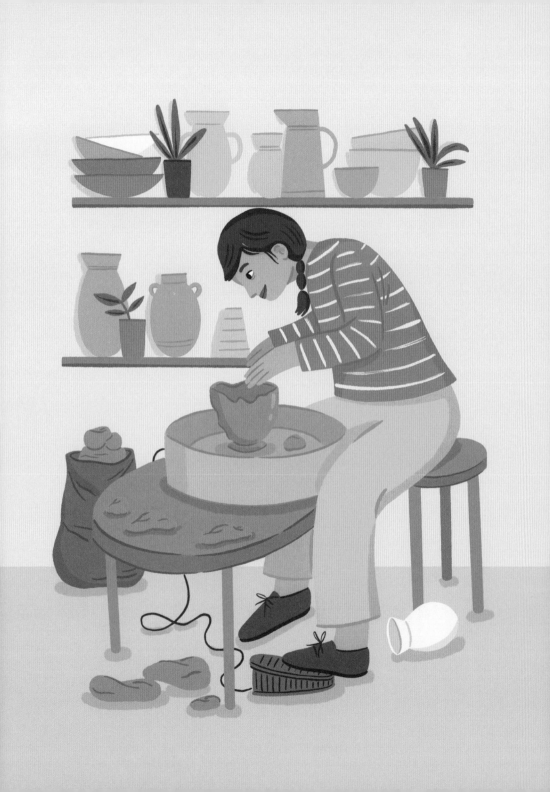

TRY THIS... **Get into Flow**

There are perhaps as many ways to enter a *flow* state as there are unique individuals. Perhaps for one person it is a sport, for another a craft, for another it is playing a particular musical instrument. Yet how do we know when we are in *flow*? What are the significant signs that we are in a *flow* experience? Psychologists on this topic tend to agree that there are six principle ways to recognise *flow*. Think of these as something of a checklist for finding and practising your own flow activities regularly. Keep in mind that while we might experience one or more of these feelings in isolation, a true *flow* experience is defined by experiencing them all simultaneously.

Checklist for flow experiences:

1. **A sense of intense focus on the present moment.**
   Young children playing are a good example of this: they exist precisely here in the moment, untaxed by future worry or bygone regrets.

2. **Awareness and activity are united.**
   If, for example, you are playing chess, the game itself will be the only thing your mind is aware of – forgetting the music playing in the distance, the twinge in your shoulder or your stomach rumbling.

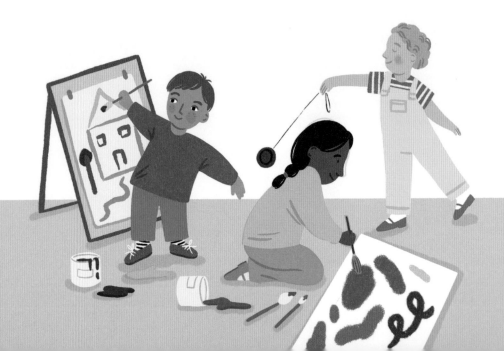

3. **A momentary loss of conscious self-awareness.**
   Similarly to the above, you will be so engrossed in the activity that
   you will 'forget yourself'.

4. **Feeling complete control over the activity.**
   You will feel just the right amount of challenge, so that you are completely
   absorbed yet completely capable – for example, you might experience
   this when swimming.

5. **Hours can pass and you do not notice.**
   You sit down in the morning to read a novel or strum away on a guitar...
   then look up at the clock and find it is suddenly past lunchtime.

6. **The activity feels rewarding in and of itself rather than a means to an end.**
   Something that you need no convincing to do and enjoy completely for its own
   sake, not to achieve another goal, e.g. Salsa dancing or singing in a choir.

Which activities cause you to experience these things? Do you have something you
do regularly that qualifies? If not, it may be time to try a new hobby to get your mind
focussed and find your *flow*.

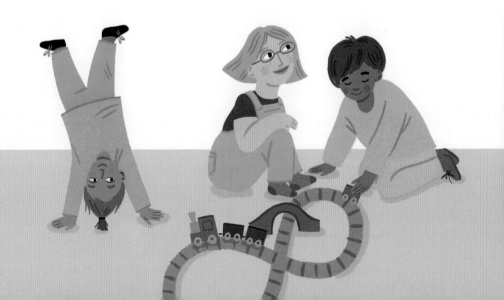

HO'OPONOPONO

həupənəupənəu | stative verb | Hawaiian
1. to put to rights; mental cleansing through forgiveness

Even with the best of intentions to stay focused, all of us will at one time or another find we stray from this path and our minds become distracted. One of the most pressing and perennial of these distractions tends to be, of course, other people – be this fall-outs with people we love or tough confrontations with colleagues. In these situations it can be harder than ever to remain mindfully serene, yet it is at such times that we may find we need this skill most of all. Perhaps this is why Hawaiians developed the concept of ho'oponopono, a practical ceremony centred around forgiveness both within and between families.

In this word, ho'o denotes cause or 'to bring about' while pono evokes order, rightness or correctness. The doubling up of pono implies 'cared for' and 'attended to' so that the combined word implies that we 'make right' or correct a situation.

Ho'oponopono illustrates a collective valuing of resolution and steadfast togetherness, offering a formal system of gathering individuals together in conference. In this indigenous forerunner of family therapy, problems can be systematically and truthfully expressed: *oia'i'o* is a key stage of the ceremony, meaning to tell the whole truth. The nine-stage ceremony also begins and closes with a prayer, which acts as an appeal for guidance from the family gods or *aumakua* and so highlights the spiritual significance of this treasured and time-honoured practice.

The cultural history of Hawaii is one characterised by change. Tragically, much of the island's indigenous culture has been warped or lost entirely. The beautiful concept of *ho'oponopono*, however, lives on and has captured the imaginations of people living far beyond this paradisiacal corner of the planet. Let it serve as a reminder to us all to stay calm, even in conflict; to let go of our gripes and experience the clean slate that arises from compassion and forgiveness.

APRAMĀDA (अ माद)

ʌ.prʌˈmaːdʌ | noun | Sanskrit
1. ethical vigilance, attentiveness or heedfulness

Around the world we have become increasingly preoccupied with the idea of mindfulness in recent years and – at least in the West – we have generally agreed upon a shared concept of this practice: to develop greater awareness of our thoughts, feelings and experiences. We have come to realise that, when we focus our attention upon the moment at hand (rather than lose ourselves in worry about the future or angst about the past), we tend to feel calmer and experience a more consistent sense of wellbeing.

It turns out, however, that there are more ways than one to be mindful of our lives and experiences. The Sanskrit term *Apramāda* (or *Appamada* in Pali) highlights a rather specific – and perhaps surprising – way to focus our minds, and an altogether different flavour of mindfulness. This form of attentiveness denotes, not just alertness to the moment as it is happening, but a manner of calm and careful vigilance over the thoughts and emotions we allow ourselves to experience, with a moral slant, similarly to the English 'prudence'.

This practice is not simply about being 'in the moment' in an ethically neutral sense, but implies that we can choose to pay close attention to the virtuousness of our thoughts, speech and actions by asking ourselves how we might have come to think the way we do. *Apramāda* therefore encourages us to ponder: what principles have we absorbed, and from where? What personal resolutions have we made, and are we living by them? Do they need updating? This draws our present attention in this moment to a calm, retrospective analysis of our past.

Complimentary to *Apramāda* is *Samprajanya* – a concept that draws our present attention towards the future, with the ultimate aim of maintaining continuity of purpose as we move through time. *Samprajanya* urges us to ask: what are our aims for the future and how are we living in alignment with these? This kind of future-focussed attentiveness may help to alter our actions in the present, promoting heightened awareness of the need to act now towards goals we may want to achieve later.

Both of these terms therefore, are as much about self-development and growth as they are about serenity in the moment. Both words are concerned not only with achieving a certain state of mind right now, but on the ways we can put attentiveness in the present moment to practical use, with the aim to live a calmer and more focussed life overall.

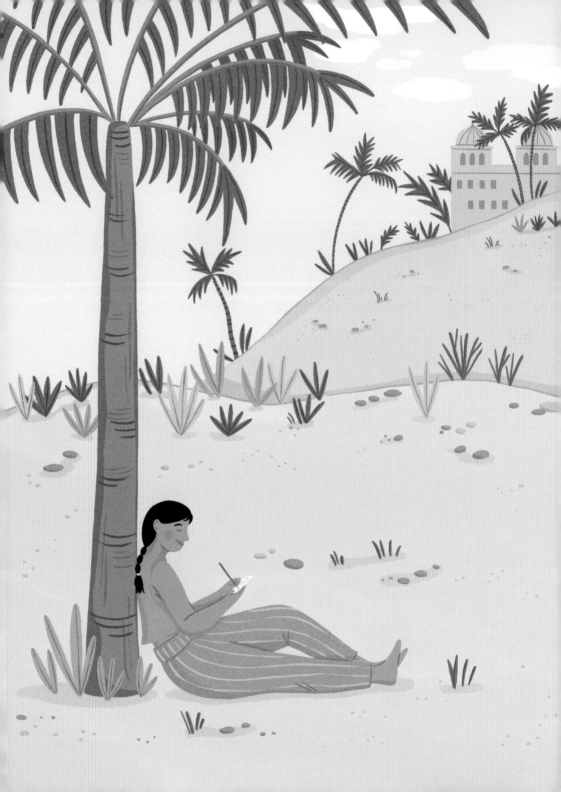

TRY THIS...

A Mindful Journal

Want to add a twist to your mindfulness practice, or start one from scratch to experience greater serenity? The Buddhist concepts of *Apramāda* and *Samprajanya* might just help. These practices have everyday benefits beyond focussing solely on the present moment. They show how making space for calm reflection upon our lives through time can help us unravel long-held assumptions from the past and to refocus our purpose as we move forward. Yet how do we realistically maintain (or even achieve) such a bird's eye view of the events of our lives?

One clever way that humans have been making sense and order out of the jumbled mass of daily experience through the ages is by keeping a diary or journal. Why might this be helpful? Well, we cannot control what we cannot measure. Therefore, it follows that if we want to gain a sense of practical control over how attentively we are living, we should keep a log – or measure – of how we are living. This is precisely what a journal can help us to do.

While it may be straightforward to establish a meditation practice to increase our awareness of the moment, this might not always help us grapple with the events and goings on of our lives as they are happening day to day. If we want to get into the habit of practising *Apramāda* and *Samprajanya*, writing down our reflections on our past and hopes for the future offers a helpful way to get started.

Perhaps you already keep a diary or journal in which you can begin to cultivate and hone the skilful attentiveness of *Apramāda* and *Samprajanya*. Or, perhaps you may wish to designate a new journal for this purpose. Either way, there is no pressure to formally grapple with these terms on the pages of your journal. Simply pose yourself these two broad questions with each entry, whatever the subject:

1. How might my past assumptions, values, experiences or decisions be affecting this present situation?

2. How might I move forward from the present situation towards my greater values and goals?

These seemingly simple questions can, over time, offer a powerful sense of our progression through the larger narrative of our lives – and help us to practise the thoughtful vigilance and purposeful continuity of *Apramāda* and *Samprajanya*.

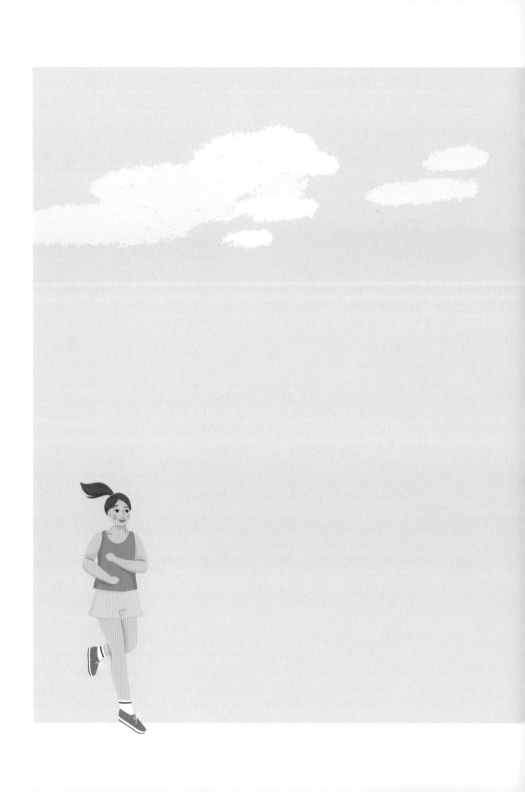

CHAPTER TWO

Body & Wellness

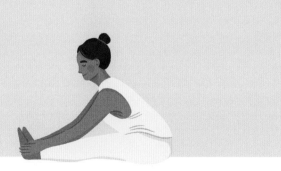

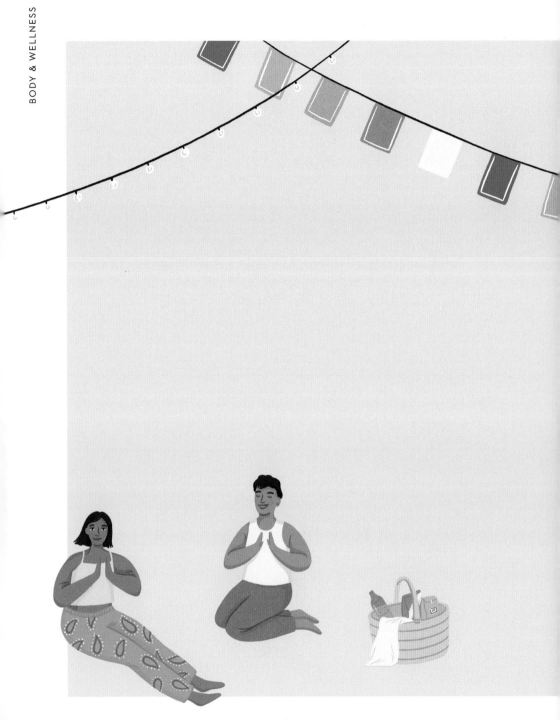

What we think affects how we feel, and vice versa. We get butterflies in our stomach when excited or nervous, sluggish when sad and upset and feel a blissful softening in our shoulders when we finally get something off our minds (or our to-do lists). These sensations illustrate the complex link between thought and physiology: our minds and bodies are not separate things. We feel our emotions in our bodies, just as what we do with our bodies can trigger emotional responses. Imagine, for example, how a hug can make us feel calmer.

As a result of this intricate mind-body relationship, we have developed many pastimes around the globe that encourage calm through physical activity. In these practices we might physically express our emotions, or simply forget our thoughts altogether in the midst of movement and feel worlds better as a result. *How* we do this around the world, however, illustrates an assortment of ways to understand the link between a well body and calm mind, and to make a regular (and enjoyable) practice of this philosophy. From communal dancing in Brazil, to the ancient breathing techniques of the yogic tradition, to the French art of strolling the city streets of Paris, to letting laughter heal us – we have invented a whole gamut of means and methods of letting our bodies do the job of working out our worries, supporting our serenity and making sense of our lives.

Perhaps there are practices and concepts here that you may already do instinctively, or perhaps there are approaches you have never before considered. Dip your toe in and discover what our world has come to know about feeling calm in both body *and* mind.

CAPOEIRA

ˌkapuˈeɪrə | noun | Portuguese (Brazil)
1. an Afro-Brazilian physical practice combining
music, dance, acrobatics and martial art

Sustained serenity is often formed of many factors, including physical and mental wellness, a sense of community support and creativity. All of these combine in the Afro-Brazilian practice of capoeira, in which large groups gather together to listen to music, sing and dance in a way that expresses the dancers' strengths, weaknesses and emotions. This physical form of self-reflection is both energising and calming.

The rich cultural history of Brazil makes it a diverse and inspiring country today, and capoeira is perhaps one of the best illustrations of this. The origins of this enchanting martial art are disputed, with some people claiming the practice originated in Brazil itself, and others arguing for its roots in African fighting techniques. Indeed, despite being widely celebrated today, capoeira has a complicated history, and was even prohibited for a time in the 19th century for its associations with street violence.

Nevertheless, the people of Brazil persevered throughout this ban by emphasising the artistic nature of the practice as a dance form, rather than its links with fighting. They were not bending the truth, either. What makes capoeira a truly unique martial art is its strong integration of music into the practice – including specific instruments such as the musical bow called a *berimbau*, and call-and-response singing styles including the *corrida* that takes place during the 'match' of two dancers. This highly creative and musical aspect serves to make capoeira a truly communal activity, reflective of Brazil's collective communal spirit (Brazil rates highly for civic participation and over 90% of Brazilians state that they would have someone to call upon in a time of need). Why not gather some friends together and head to a capoeira class near you?

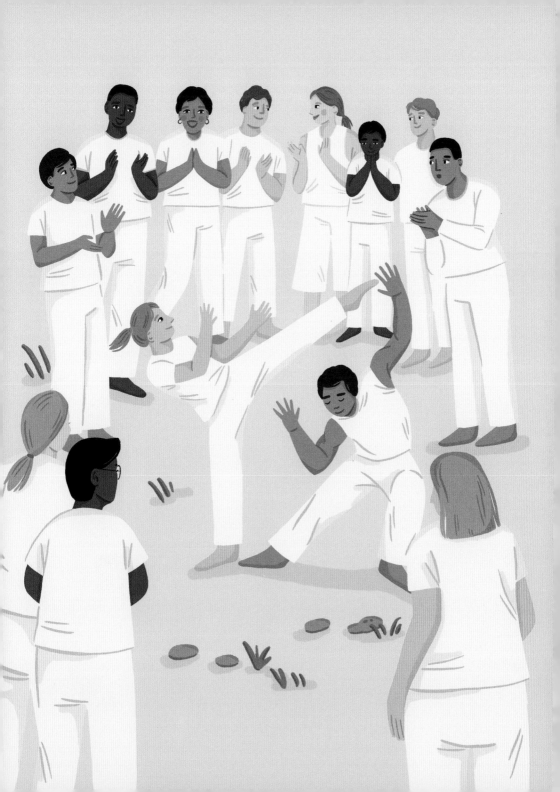

TRY THIS...

Stretch it out, Capoeira style

To benefit from the calming effects of *capoeira* there are a number of stretches you can try that are influenced by the style. These are gentle, sweeping moves that should be done slowly as a warm up (avoid any sudden moves). Take extra care if you have any existing injuries and always check with a professional if you have concerns.

1. Lie on your back and take a few deep breaths. Keep up this focussed breathing throughout your stretches.

2. Turn slightly to lie on one side and, ensuring that your abdominal muscles are engaged, sweep the top leg around in large sweeping circles. Repeat three times and then swap sides.

3. Do a similar circular motion, but this time with your arm. Repeat three circular sweeps before swapping sides to complete with the other arm.

4. From here, roll onto your tummy and use your arms to lift your torso off the floor in the style of a cobra. Hold for a few breaths and then lift up onto your hands

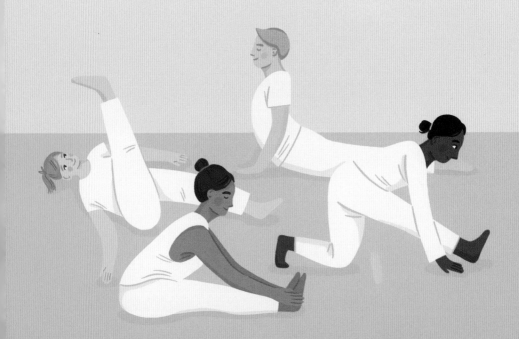

and feet, keeping your back and legs as straight as possible, in an upside-down V shape. Hold this for a few breaths.

5. Sit back onto the floor with your legs stretched apart (as wide as comfortable). Place your palms on the floor in front of you and lean gently forward until you can feel the stretch in your thighs and legs. Take a few slow breaths here.

6. Lift your hands over your head and take your torso over towards your right foot, breathing into the stretch (you should feel it along the left side of your body). After a few breaths, repeat on the opposite side.

7. Bring your legs together so that they stretch out straight in front of you. Lift your arms in the air and then down to touch your toes. Breathe into this stretch for a few moments, and then release to gently roll down and lie on your back once again (lifting your knees so your feet are on the floor will make this roll-down easier on your back). Once lying down, take a few slow breaths here, noticing how your body feels after these stretches.

8. If you can, finish your practice with a classic 'crab' move by lifting up onto your hands and feet from your lying position and holding this for a few breaths.

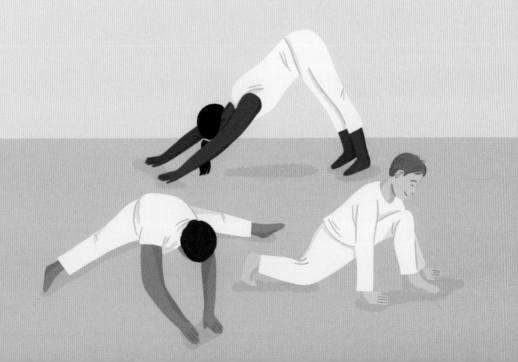

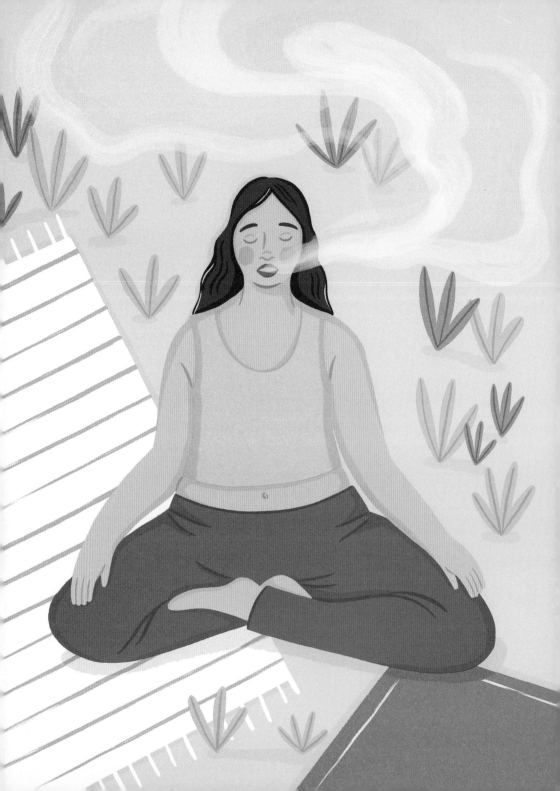

PRĀṆĀYĀMA (प्राणायाम)

ˌprɑːnʌˈjɑːmə: | noun | Sanskrit
1. breath control

All humans around the world rely on their breath to live. This simple, persistent, non-negotiable aspect of our existence (and, of course, our physical wellbeing) can nevertheless get somewhat forgotten. How often are you aware of your breath? Perhaps not often. Yet we ignore this essential facet of our wellness at our own peril given that the breath is something of a barometer for how calm - or stressed - we are in a given moment.

On a particularly stressful day, we might catch our selves holding our breath with frustration, or breathing in a very shallow way. We might even notice that we let out sudden, weary sighs seemingly from nowhere, or that our breath becomes short and panicked. In fact, the breath is not only a way of measuring our physical state, but actually of affecting how well we feel. Certain breathing techniques can calm us, energise, help us focus, help us fall asleep and much more - and this is exactly what is captured by the branch of yoga known as *Prāṇāyāma* (breath control).

While in the West we might be forgiven for associating yoga purely with *Asana* (posture); *Prāṇāyāma* is equally fundamental to yogic philosophy. In fact, yoga originated in ancient India as an outline for an entire system of physical, mental and spiritual wellness - not merely as an adjunct form of exercise.

Prāṇāyāma is a Sanskrit term - formed of *prāna* meaning 'breath' or 'vital force' and *āyāma* meaning 'restraint' or 'control'. It elevates breathing from everyday, ubiquitous, almost-accidental necessity into an art form that is under our control, and which we can wield to great benefit.

Prāṇāyāma comes in many forms, but is usually composed of three parts. These are: *Purak* (inhalation), *Kumbhak* (retention) and *Rechak* (exhalation). *Prāṇāyāma* can be practised alone or in combination with yogic postures.

The purpose of controlling our breath in this way is to experience greater rejuvenation and restoration from our breathing. What is wonderful about this practice is its simplicity - wherever we are, we can attend to our breath to instantly calm or revive ourselves.

TRY THIS... **Ocean Breath**

Ujjayi Prānāyāma – sometimes colloquially known as 'Ocean Breath' because of the sound it makes, which can be likened to the rushing waves of the ocean – is an especially calming breathing practice. This is similar to a kind of breathing that we all already do and recognise: the kind that occurs just as we nod off to sleep. If you have ever seen someone drop off in an armchair or beside you on the train, then you will be able to distinguish this kind of breathing. It catches softly in the throat, almost like a gentle snore, making a raspy sound like rushing water. As this is the kind of breathing we do naturally when we sleep, it is considered especially restorative and soothing. You can give *Ujjayi Prānāyāma* a go whenever you need a moment of serenity, or when you feel that five minutes of focussed breathing might offer you some added calm – such as before a big meeting or at bedtime.

Tips for getting started with *Ujjayi* breathing*

1. To begin, find a quiet place to assume a comfortable seated position, either cross-legged on the floor or comfortably in a chair.

2. Close your eyes and let your mouth gently open. Begin to notice the rhythm of your natural breathing.

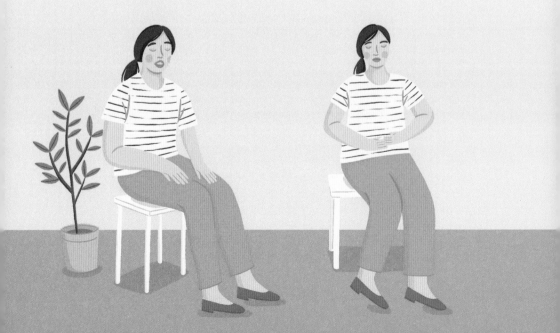

3. When ready, on your out-breath imagine you are fogging up a window and let out a soft, raspy 'ahh' – like the rush of an ocean wave.

4. Repeat this several times: breathing in as normal and out with Ocean Breath.

5. Let your in-breath expand deeply into your belly (but keep in mind that in order to stay comfortable and avoid any light-headedness, you will want to breathe in until just before your lungs feel at capacity, and out until just before they feel empty).

6. There is no need to count the breath – just work with your own natural rhythm.

7. If it is comfortable, after some time allow your mouth to close so that you are inhaling and exhaling from the nose, but still maintaining the throaty, ocean sound on the out-breath. Continue for five minutes.

This introductory practice focuses on the *Ujjayi* out-breath, as it is easier than the in-breath. After some practise, for full *Ujjayi Prānāyāma*, you may wish to add in the in-breath with the same smooth, steady rushing sound (this can take a lot of practise!).

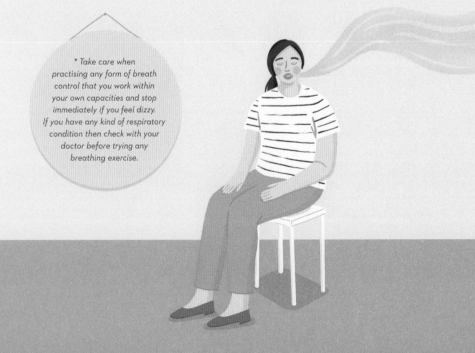

* Take care when practising any form of breath control that you work within your own capacities and stop immediately if you feel dizzy. If you have any kind of respiratory condition then check with your doctor before trying any breathing exercise.

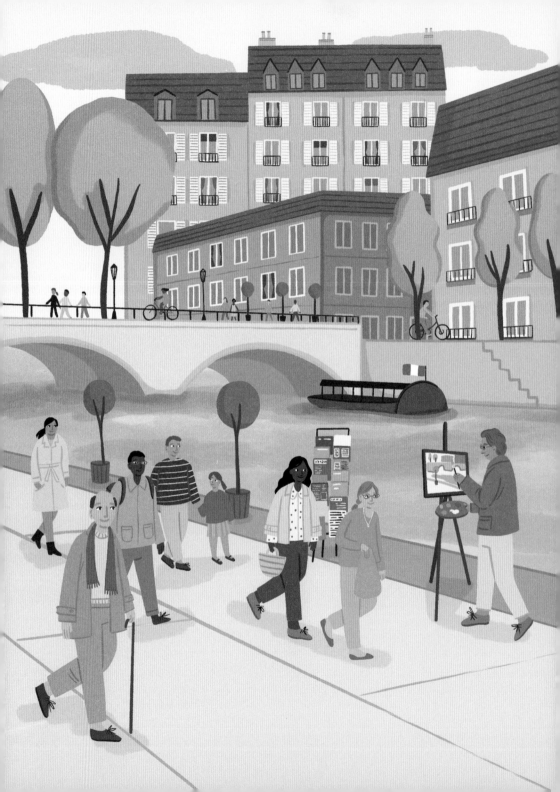

FLÂNEUR

flanœʀ | noun (m.) | French
1. a man who strolls leisurely around while observing society

The humble stroll – known rather fittingly in antiquated English as a
'constitutional' – truly does wonders to improve our physical wellbeing.
From aiding digestion to clearing our minds, there is not much a good
walk cannot help with – and that includes helping us to feel more serene.

There are many different ways that we enjoy the calming effects of
a good walk around the world. The Dutch people relish *uitwaaien* (to
walk in the wind for fun), while the Greeks enjoy a traditional *volta*
(stroll along the shore or main street at sundown), and the English like
rambling (walking in the countryside for pleasure). Yet perhaps one of
the most studied and sophisticated of these ways of enjoying a walk
is the character of the *flâneur*: a French masculine noun referring to a
'saunterer' or 'loafer' that is synonymous with bygone artists, scholars
and literary figures of Paris who would wander the city and observe
its goings-on. More recently, you can also find the term *flâneuse* – the
female equivalent.

These terms originate from the slightly less sophisticated French
term *flânerie*, meaning aimless or idle behaviour, and yet have been
elevated over time to reflect an activity that is both quintessentially
Parisian and yet recognisable behaviour to anyone who has spent
time in a metropolitan city: 'people watching' as one soaks up the
urban atmosphere.

What is lovely about this term is that it highlights how moving our
bodies for greater serenity and wellbeing need not require that we live
in a countryside idyll or take regular weekend trips to the mountains. We
can benefit from the calming effects of a daily walk simply by relishing in
what our external environment *does* have to offer. In fact, the figure of
the *flâneur* or *flâneuse* celebrates the specific pleasure of strolling in a
metropolitan environment because we can soak up the unique and varied
sights, sounds and inspiration offered by these spaces.

If you are a city-dweller, take your own urban stroll today and notice
the relaxing effects of observing and revelling in the inner-city sphere.

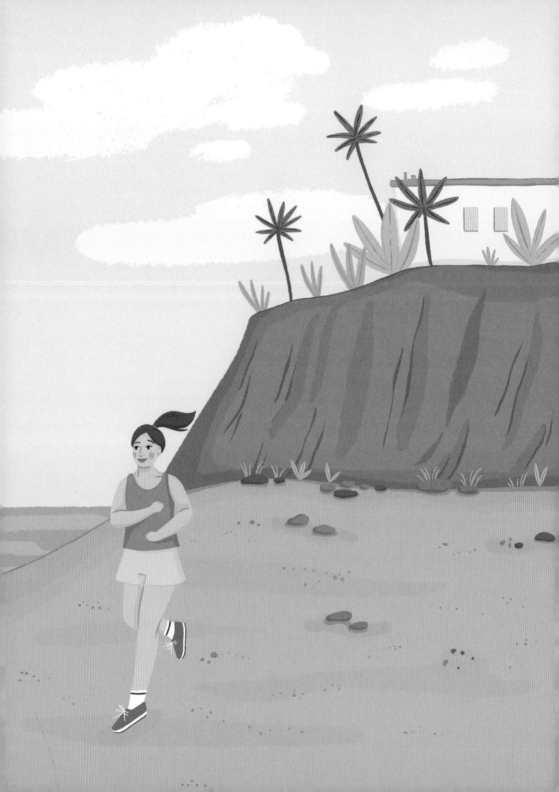

DESABAFÁR

ʤɪzəbæsa: | verb | Portuguese
1. to take some fresh air; to vent

Our feelings of stress are intimately tied with our physical environments, and English speakers use many physical analogies to evoke our emotions. We might exclaim that we feel figuratively 'trapped' or 'stuck', or that our emotions are 'weighing on us'. This feeling of heaviness or stuck-ness can be overcome in many ways: sometimes by talking to others or writing things down in a journal. Sometimes, though, our minds are helped by quite literally giving our selves 'breathing space': by getting outside and moving around. All of these ways that we 'vent' or 'unburden' ourselves are captured in the interesting Portuguese verb *desabafár*.

Desabafár means anything from getting something 'off our chest' by sharing it in conversation, to 'letting off steam' by physically going for a run. This is a word that does a wonderful job of illustrating the close links between our minds and our physical bodies: a revitalising run in the fresh air can feel just as good as telling a friend our troubles, and vice versa. When we move our bodies, we often process our emotions as effectively as we might have in talking them through – perhaps, at times, more effectively.

Interestingly, *desabafár* has its etymological roots in the word *abafar* (suffocate), so the suggestion of the term is that one is 'de-suffocating' oneself either by getting outside or unburdening oneself of a secret. There is, therefore, something distinctly Portuguese about *desabafár* and its description of freeing ourselves of troubling emotions. The people of Portugal are famous for their lamenting *fado* music, which expresses sadness and *saudade* (longing) through the medium of song. What *desabafár* highlights is that – while singing or discussing our woes in words might be marvellously helpful, getting outside and moving our bodies can be an equally effective way to process and dispel stress.

Next time you find yourself feeling 'stifled' or 'suffocated' by feelings of stress, try to *desabafár* (unburden) yourself by getting outside in the fresh air; allowing your body to process whatever is troubling your mind. It may just work wonders.

HÓZHÓ

hɒʒəu | noun | Navajo
1. a philosophy of wellness through balanced living

Some terms and concepts are so rich with meaning that it is almost impossible to appreciate them outside of their culture and language of usage. Such is the case with the *Hózhó* philosophy of the Diné (Navajo) people, which implies a combination of 'balance', 'harmony', 'health', 'wholeness', 'resilience' and 'beauty'.

Diné Bikéyah, or Navajoland, covers over twenty-seven thousand square miles crossing the states of Utah, New Mexico and Arizona – and for the people of this nation *Hózhó* promotes a way of being that is conducive to a long and healthy existence. This arises through taking pride in one's thoughts, actions, physical body and spirit. It also involves cultivating a reverence for all forms of life on Earth, in a way that fosters good interpersonal relationships with others.

What makes *Hózhó* a particularly complex word to grasp is that it evokes both a state of being and a way of living, or a set of behaviours. More than this, it covers a vast array of positive qualities, all of which one might expect to find in someone who fully modelled *Hózhó* such as a well-respected Diné elder. This could include any number of positive qualities, but of particular interest is the physical discipline that *Hózhó* celebrates. Meticulous self-respect, self-care and physical activity are paramount to living in alignment with the *Hózhó* model.

Of course, the idea that physical strength and wellness would be valuable to a people that were historically hunter-gathers, reliant on sustained team effort to thrive, is obvious. Yet what might this mean in the modern day? Staying physically strong through a regular routine of healthy habits and exercise can keep us calm and well for *ourselves*, but also helps us to be there in support of *others*. If our health and serenity fail, we lack the strength and peace of mind to support others – and this idea is central to *Hózhó*. This concept offers a gentle reminder, then, that physical self-care is not self-centred, but part of being a good member of our community.

TAKE A DIP...
WAYS WE BATHE

Across the globe we have a special relationship with water and bathing. For many of us, few things better inspire calm and rejuvenation than a hot steamy soak in a tub, perhaps accompanied by beautifully fragranced bath oils, candlelight and music. Naturally, however, even something as seemingly straightforward as a dip (in the bath, in a pool or in another context) has been imagined and re-imagined by different cultures and languages around the world.

Ayurveda is the classic Hindu method of medicine based around the idea of balancing bodily systems through herbal treatments, food and breathing techniques. In this tradition, bathing is considered a healing and sacred activity. Ancient Ayurvedic texts reportedly advise elaborate therapeutic baths incorporating milk, honey, rose petals and even turmeric. In fact, *snana* (bathing) forms a vital facet of *dinacharya* (the 'daily routine' in Ayurveda), along with other essential activities like *udvartana* (massage) and *dantadhavana* (cleaning teeth).

While a warm bath with rose petals might sound like an instantly appealing remedy, in many of the colder climes of the world quite the opposite is encouraged as a benefit to health: cold-water swimming. In the North of Scotland, parts of Scandinavia, Russia and North America this sport is increasingly practised by a legion of enthusiastic fans – and they might be onto something. Some initial studies have suggested that exposure to cold water, for example a cold shower, could be helpful for those suffering with depression. This is because intense cold is known to activate the sympathetic nervous system and increase blood levels of beta-endorphin (primarily utilised in the body to reduce stress).

If a dip – hot or cold – is not your thing, then how about a steam? In South Sudan, married women (or women preparing for marriage) may participate in a *dukhan*, in which the body is rubbed with scented oils, wrapped in a blanket and 'smoked' over a pit of aromatic wood. Elsewhere, across Mexico and Central America, you may enjoy a *temazcal*. This is a cave-like structure utilised much like a sweat lodge to cleanse the body, as well as to spiritually reflect. Applying aloe vera, mud or herbs to the body during a *temazcal* ceremony is also common.

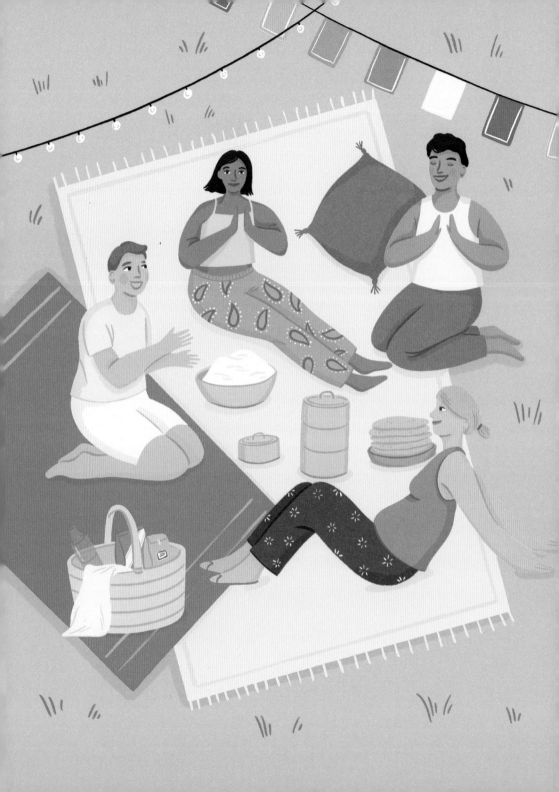

HASYA YOGA

ɦɑːs.jɑː joː.gɑː | Practice | India and USA
1. laughter yoga

When we are feeling stressed there are some obvious go-to things we might do in order to calm down and feel better. We might take a long bath, meditate or chat things through with a friend over a glass of wine... but what about having a good old belly laugh?

One of the best stress-busters we have built in is laughter. Yet laughing might feel like the last thing we want to do when frazzled by life's demands. Typically we think that laughter requires a source: something that is rib-achingly funny, like a stand-up comic or hilarious movie. Yet the practice of *hasya yoga* tells a different story. This practice was established by the Indian medical doctor and guru of giggling Dr Madan Kataria in the mid 1990s, and has since spread to the USA and worldwide. *Hasya* in Sanskrit translates into English as 'humour' or 'comedy'. *Hasya yoga* is based upon the reasoning that, after about thirty seconds, the body cannot make a physiological distinction between real, spontaneous laughter and phony or imitated laughter. Because of this, teachers of *hasya yoga* contend, we will get the same physical benefits either way. Added to that is the fact that an insincere chuckle can often result in a genuine bout of the giggles – especially when we try this practice with a group of others.

What are the benefits of laughter? Well, firstly laughter releases tension – hence why we often laugh when nervous or in an uncomfortable situation. More than this, a recent study published in *The Journal of Neuroscience* found that the feel-good endorphins released during bouts of social laughter not only trigger pleasurable feelings and relieve pain but also support both the formation and reinforcement of social bonds. This euphoric mix of happy hormones and social closeness is a winning combination for feeling calmer, and for replacing anxiety with both an immediate and long-lasting boost to our wellbeing. Do you need any more convincing of the feel-good effects of a giggle?

TRY THIS...

Hasya Yoga Warm Up and Exercises

While children reportedly laugh on average three to four hundred times *per day*, for adults it is closer to a mere ten to fifteen times – and many of these grown-up sniggers come in the form of polite social laughter rather than the genuinely elated hilarity of childhood. Is there a link between our increased anxiety in adulthood and our apparent tendency to take ourselves so seriously? Perhaps. Early research into the benefits of *hasya yoga* has indicated that these may include both reduced blood pressure and a reduction of stress hormones in the blood including cortisol. One thing is for sure: we have little to lose by introducing a bit more laughter into our lives, and perhaps a lot to gain. A fundamental aspect of the practice of *hasya yoga* is the social connection and 'contagious' laughter that comes from giggling with others, so grab a friend or two and give these exercises a go. Fifteen minutes is ideal, but you may enjoy yourself so much that you will lose track of time and get into some genuine snickering... If you feel absolutely daft doing these exercises, then you are doing them right!

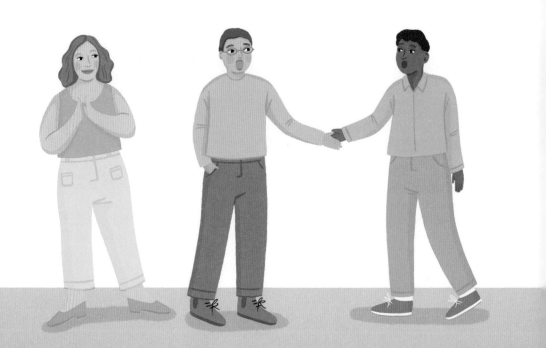

Getting started

To begin, try the typical warm up of a *hasya yoga* session. Clap your hands together and chant 'Ho Ho, Ha Ha Ha' several times, while making eye contact with other members in your group. You might find that this alone gets you into a fit of giggles. As you try the different exercises below, return to this clapping exercise between each one in order to structure the practice and calm you down if things get too hyper.

Greeting laughter

In this exercise, you move around the room and shake hands with the group, continuing to make eye contact and to repeat your 'Ho Ho, Ha Ha Ha' chant. If you are giving this a go with just one friend, you might like to try simply alternating hands as you shake.

Phone laughter

Here, you hold your hand to your ear imitating a phone call and pretend that you are speaking to someone who has just said something extremely funny (you might like to imagine a particularly funny friend). Imitate big belly laughs as you do this.

Silent laughter

Have you ever experienced the desire to laugh in a wholly inappropriate situation, and had to laugh silently? If so, you will know that the need to be silent can increase hilarity. Try laughing quietly, without making a sound, and see how you do.

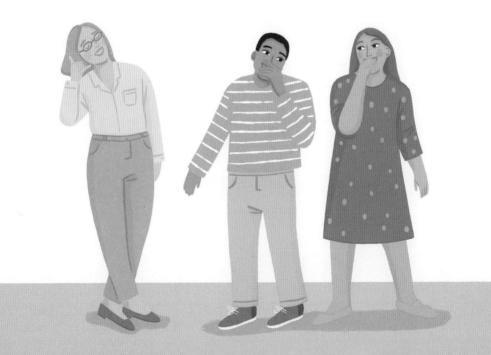

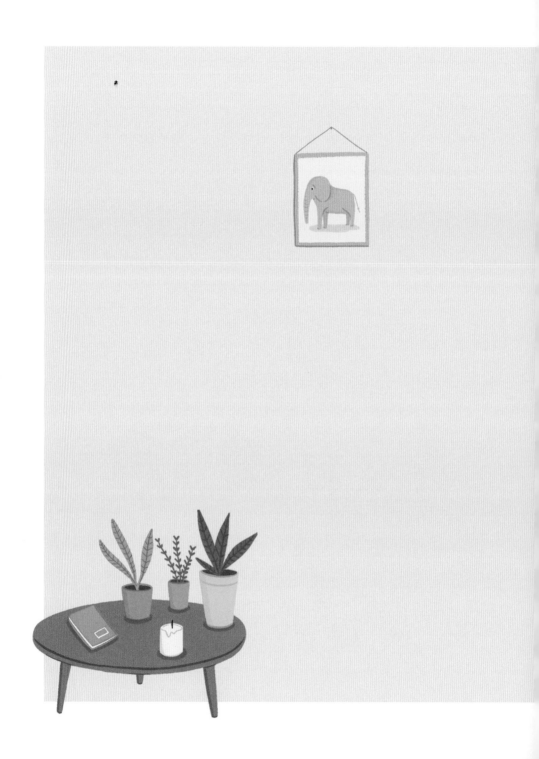

CHAPTER THREE

Habits & Rituals

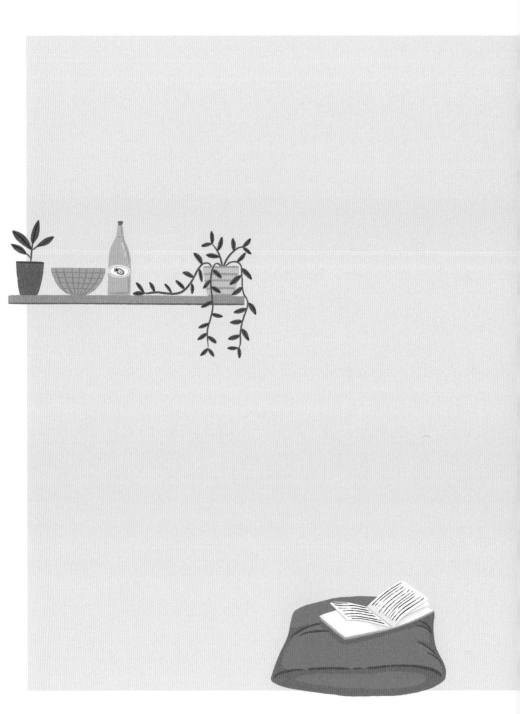

To take the stress out of de-stressing, it can be useful to establish a regular, non-negotiable habit. It is reassuring to have regular habits that are non-negotiable, perhaps simply because we do not have to labour over these decisions and thus they make life feel easier. This chapter is all about the kinds of habits that keep us calm, well and give us an opportunity to slow down so that we can prioritise what is important to us. Around the world we do just this with everyday rituals that keep us calm and connected to others.

What constitutes a calming habit, of course, varies widely around our globe. Across our many different nations and cultures we gravitate time and again to certain blissful rituals and traditions that help us relax and feel content. Sometimes a seasonal change brings with it certain customs that we anticipate the rest of the year. Or, we make a daily ritual out of something as simple as our coffee break at work. Elsewhere we make a habit of helping others by performing regular good deeds that help us feel connected to our community. In many places we watch as our whole community slows down once per week on a Sunday.

Whether you already have treasured rituals that keep you feeling calm and connected, or are in search of a few more, this chapter explores some clever ways that different cultures have evolved to keep a measure of calm in their daily, weekly and even yearly routines. You may not adopt them all – perhaps just one or two will inspire you to start a relaxing new ritual in your own life – but they will all teach you something about the culture in which they originate. What are you waiting for? Get in the habit of serene living today.

FIKA

/'fiːˌka/ | noun | Swedish
1. a coffee break as a social activity, often with sweet-baked goods

Even the busiest day will benefit from a break in proceedings to refuel, grab some downtime and catch up with friends. If we do not take time to rest, then the remainder of our time tends to be less productive – because it is in our break time that we re-energise for activities to come. These pauses in our day serve as the punctuation marks around our productivity, helping us catch our breath in an otherwise non-stop revolving door of duties and tasks.

One culture that has raised the ritual of the midday coffee break to new heights is Swedish culture where we find the practice of *fika*. This word stems from a trend in Sweden in the 19th century to use back slang (the inversion of syllables in words) so that *kaffi* or 'coffee' became *fika*. Yet this term has come to imply much more than just a beverage; it denotes a beloved daily ritual (and sometimes twice or three times daily!) of pausing to sit down and catch up with others over a warm drink and a sweet treat.

This word can be used as both a noun and a verb. You could say that you would like to have *fika*, but you might also ask someone 'want to *fika*?'. Either way, this is a habit that is much-loved by all Swedes. *Fika* can happen whether at home, at work or out and about in a café. What is most endearing about this word is the way it speaks to the joy Swedish people take in the simple pleasures of life: even the humble coffee break. While coffee in many other cultures is a hurried affair, sipped while standing at a counter or taken in a to-go cup on the way to the next meeting, *fika* makes coffee an opportunity to relish our break time so that this simple necessity of life – the mid-morning or mid-afternoon refuel – can be savoured and enjoyed collectively.

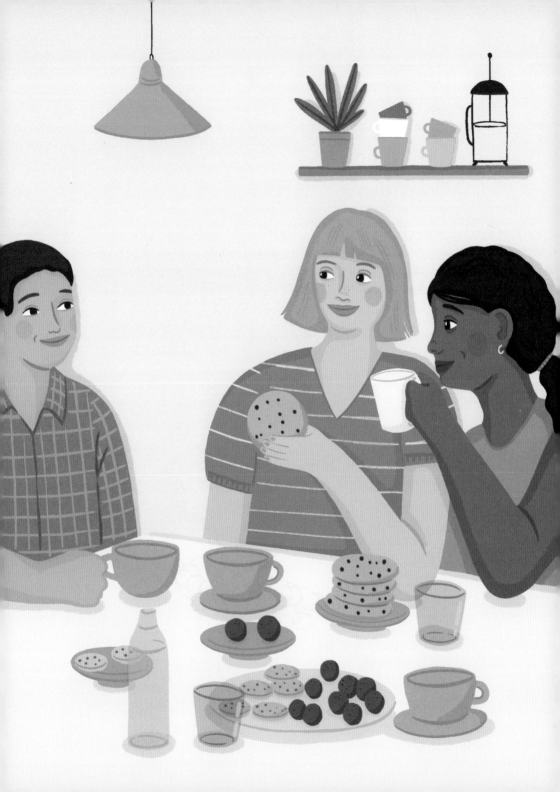

TRY THIS...

Cinnamon Buns

Aside from coffee, nothing is more synonymous with *fika* in Sweden than the cinnamon bun. The indulgent warmth of this sweet treat goes perfectly with a hot drink, whether morning or afternoon.

Try out this recipe for an authentic Swedish *fika* experience.

Makes 35 buns

50g fresh yeast
150g butter
250ml milk
250ml water
2 eggs
130g caster sugar
1 tablespoon ground cardamom
½ teaspoon salt
800g plain flour

FOR THE CINNAMON FILLING:
(NB these amounts can be doubled for
*   extra cinnamon goodness!)*
150g butter
850g caster sugar
1 tablespoon ground cinnamon
1 egg

TO GARNISH:
1 egg whisked, for brushing
50g pearl sugar (*pärlsocker* in Swedish)

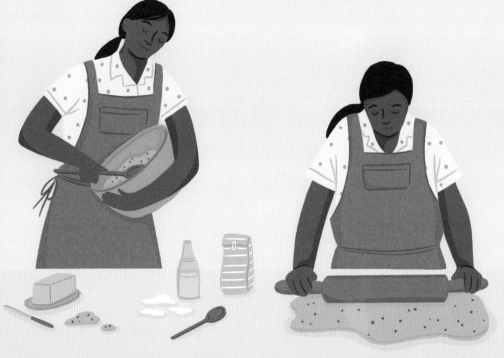

Method

1. Put the yeast in a large mixing bowl.

2. Melt the butter and then add the milk and water. This mixture needs to be about 37°C (98°F) so you may want to warm the milk and water slightly. Pour the mixture over the yeast and stir until the yeast dissolves.

3. Add the eggs, sugar, cardamom, salt and almost all of the flour (save some for the rolling).

4. Work into dough until it stops sticking to the edges of the mixing bowl. If it seems a little too wet at this stage, you may want to add some extra flour. Cover the bowl with a tea towel and leave to rise for 40 minutes.

5. While the dough is rising, prepare the filling by mixing together the butter, sugar and cinnamon. Line one or two baking trays with baking paper.

6. Transfer the dough to a floured kitchen surface. If it still seems a little too wet at this stage, work in a little extra flour until you have a soft springy dough. Using a floured rolling pin, make one (or two) large rectangles. Spread the filling onto the dough. Roll the dough together and slice into 35 pieces, around 2cm thick.

7. Shape the slices into rounds directly onto your baking trays. Cover with a tea towel and leave the buns to rise for a further 30 minutes. Preheat the oven to 250°C/Gas 8.

8. Brush the buns with the whisked egg and sprinkle the pearl sugar on top. Bake the buns in the middle of the oven for 8–10 minutes and then cool on a wire rack. Then, enjoy!

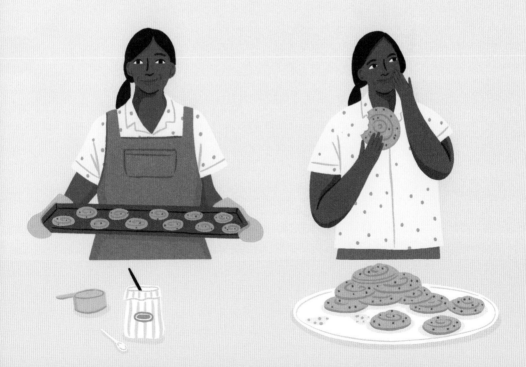

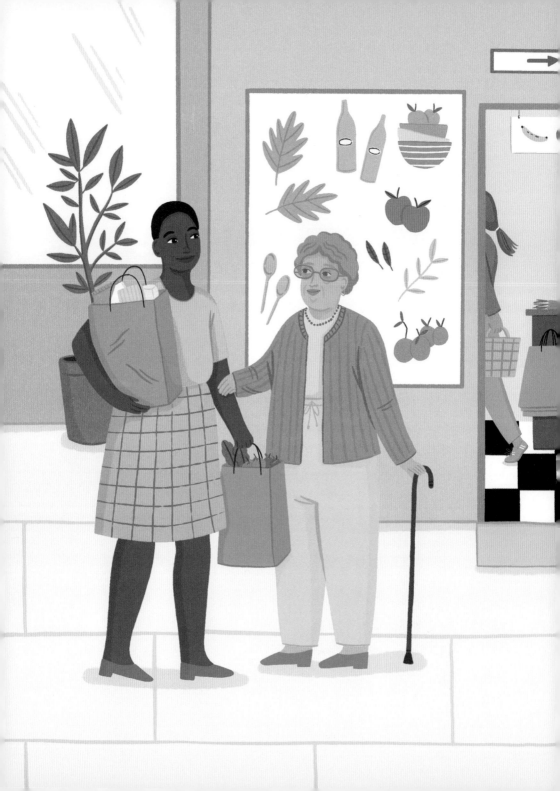

MITZVAH (מִצְוָה)

'mɪtsvə | noun | Hebrew
1. a good deed or moral act

When it comes to habits that are conducive to serenity, we might imagine ourselves cross-legged in meditation, solitary and detached from the hubbub of daily reality. Yet the truth is that most moments of our lives do not look like this. We live among others: in partnerships, families, communities and cultures, wherein – to thrive as a whole – we need to all get along and support a certain collective calm. What might it mean to keep our communal cool, then, and what are the kinds of habits that support this? The humble art of the good deed, or *mitzvah* in Hebrew, is a good place to start.

To do a *mitzvah*, in modern liberal usage of the term, is to perform a kind act for another person. The literal translation of *mitzvah* is 'commandment', yet the idea of being simply commanded or obligated to perform such a kind deed does not do this term justice. Doing a *mitzvah* suggests wholehearted sincerity in the act. While the word is bound up with duty, it is also one of compassionate sentiment and the genuine aspiration to feel connected to others; a *mitzvah* is valuable in itself, not merely a means to an end.

The popular idea of 'self-care' is a welcomed antidote if we spend our lives in service of others, but if we notice that we *rarely* act generously, then cultivating this habit of kindness will support not only the wellbeing of others, but also our own in turn. One recent study found that performing kind acts for others resulted in improved mood among those with social anxiety, perhaps in part because of the reassuring sense of community we build when we act this way.

The truth is that staying calm is not always about ritualistically isolating ourselves in meditative repose, but instead can include the creation of habits that help us feel affinity with others. There is the old saying that there is strength in numbers; so too, as the *mitzvah* concept suggests, is there serenity in numbers.

MUSIC TO OUR EARS...
THE HARMONY OF SONG

There are all manner of distinct calming habits and rituals found around the world, from sources as varied as built-up contemporary cities, centuries-old religions and more nomadic cultures living close to nature. A shared ritual we find across practically all of these diverse communities and cultures, however, is the practice of music – whether that be rhythmic drumming, choirs, jam sessions, rap battles or even elaborate orchestral concertos. Music provides us with solace in troubled times, brings us together with others and restores our spirits.

Even in largely secular societies, music has the power to make us feel we transcend ourselves. Standing in the crowd of a music festival, or sitting in the stalls of a classical concert, or even singing in a small group of others are all opportunities for elevation beyond the individual sense of self (a rare experience in individualistic societies). Music unites and heartens us, and in this it also has the power to bring us a great sense of peace and tranquility.

In West Africa we find the practice of *djembe* drumming. In Bambara language, *djé* means 'to gather' and *bé* means 'peace', and so this rhythmic ritual implies that to drum together is to find solidarity and tranquillity among others. From ancient Sanskrit is the art of *kirtan*

(कीर्तन) chanting. The term *kirtan* means to tell or to describe an idea or story, and *kirtan* chanting often involves a kind of call-and-response between a group of chanters sharing a legend or spiritual narrative, accompanied by a range of musical instruments.

Around the world, poetry – often set to music – also offers us a sense of serenity. Again in Sanskrit we find the term *bhakti* (भक्ति), which literally means 'devotion' and implies intense personal worship of a supreme deity that has traditionally been expressed through deeply emotional and celebrant poetry. *Doină*, from Romania, is a form of traditional lyrical poetry not unlike the elegy of classical Greek and Latin literature, which allows for the cathartic expression of joy and sadness, love and loneliness and all the human experiences in between.

Across Kenya, Tanzania and on the island of Zanzibar we find the *taarab* style of music, characterised by its jubilant blending of the musical traditions of Africa, the Middle East and the Indian Subcontinent. *Taarab* is a word loaned from Arabic, meaning 'having joy with music'. Indeed, through both music and poetry we each have and experience all manner of emotions. In this beautiful outlet of our inner feelings, we share and connect with one another, and find tremendous reassurance and peace.

UTEPILS

u:tepɪls | noun | Norwegian
1. drinking a beer outside with friends

We remark on the changing of seasons as we gradually notice alterations in the weather – such as lighter evenings in the summertime or the chill in the air that comes with autumn. We also mark these seasonal changes with key rituals that we collectively associate with these seasons. In hot weather we might relax around the barbecue, while winter is a time for cosier indoor gatherings, perhaps around the fire in a good country pub. What these rituals highlight is how – come rain or shine, and across myriad cultures – we find ways to relax together.

In Norway, we find a term that perfectly captures this spirit of the seasonally specific ritual, and of the internationally revered pastime of sharing a drink with our friends: *utepils*. This is the name given to a beer that we drink outside because the weather is fine, but the

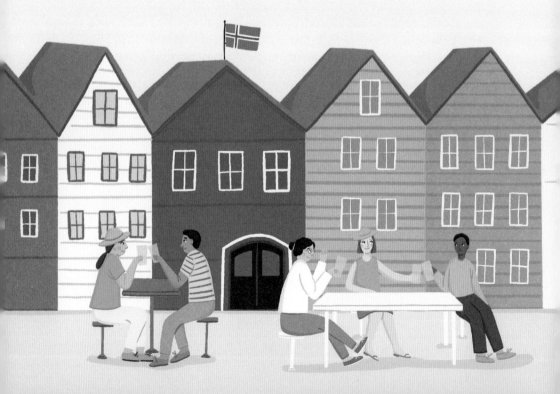

term particularly evokes the anticipation of the *first* beer that can be appreciated outside following a Norwegian winter.

This endearing term is compounded from two words: *ute*, which literally means 'outside', and *pils*, which is simply short for Pilsner – a popular beer in the country. For Norwegians, there are few signs of the springtime that are more recognised or celebrated than when the temperature raises just enough to allow everybody to once again congregate in beer gardens – even if lap blankets are required – to share a beer with friends.

The pleasure taken in something so seemingly minor – venturing out of doors for a drink – is understandable when you consider that this is a nation where winters are bitterly cold. Temperatures can drop as low as minus 40°C in some parts of the country. Winter nights in Norway are also disproportionately long and, in the very northern part of this nation, the sun does not rise at all through winter. Relaxing outside after one of these winters therefore must feel like an extraordinary treat, and is one that Norwegians revisit year upon year with ritualistic zeal.

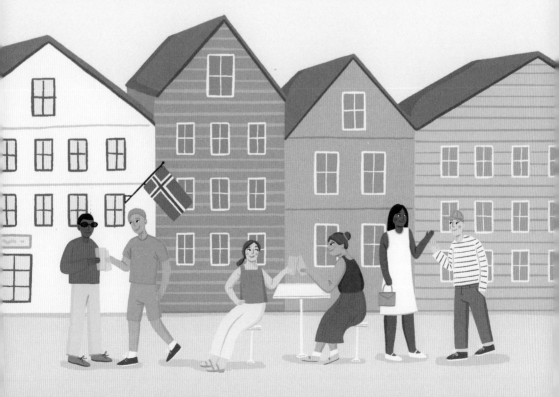

DOMINGUEAR

dɒmɪŋgeɪɑ: | verb | Spanish

1. to partake in activities associated with Sunday

There are many daily rituals and seasonal habits that we associate with calm around the world. Yet what about that regular weekly occasion where many of us take the opportunity to relax? Sunday. Long considered to be the 'day of rest' in many cultures, lots of us associate Sundays with having little on our plates, taking the chance to rest and putting our feet up. Rather wonderfully, in Spain and parts of Latin America, there is a slang word in the form of a verb to precisely capture the spirit of this day: *dominguear*. This term stems from *Domingo*, meaning Sunday, and creates a verb form out of it: 'to Sunday', or to do an activity associated with the day (you might also hear *domingueando*, or 'Sunday-ing').

The use of *dominguear* can be context specific depending on what activities you and yours associate with Sunday – which, for many, is

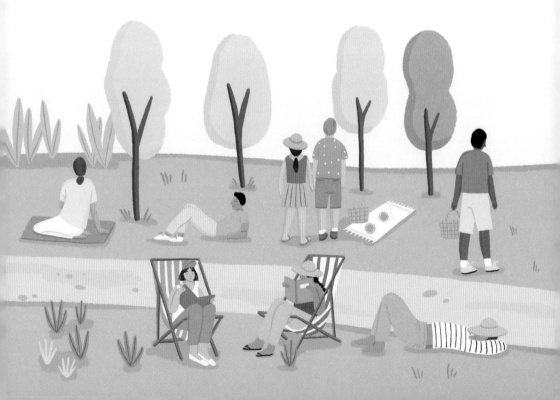

a religious day. If you are a church-going family then *dominguear* might imply putting on your 'Sunday best' (your smartest clothes) and heading off to church. Yet for those that do not actively attend church, *domingueando* is all about pausing, going slowly and taking a breather out of your busy week. This term is so associated with slowing down that in some countries such as Argentina it is even possible to pejoratively refer to someone as a *dominguero* if they drive too slowly, i.e. they are a 'Sunday driver'.

Although *dominguear* is not found in all Spanish-speaking nations, it is nevertheless a charming concept that captures the ritualistic slowing down that is synonymous with Sunday. At the end of a busy week we can all benefit from taking a breather to rest, relax, dawdle a little and generally behave in a more leisurely manner. Why not take the opportunity yourself and invite the habit of *domingueando* into your week. This weekend, clear your schedule and commit to the considered art of Sunday-ing: taking the time to pause, like a relaxed in-breath before the busyness starts up again come Monday.

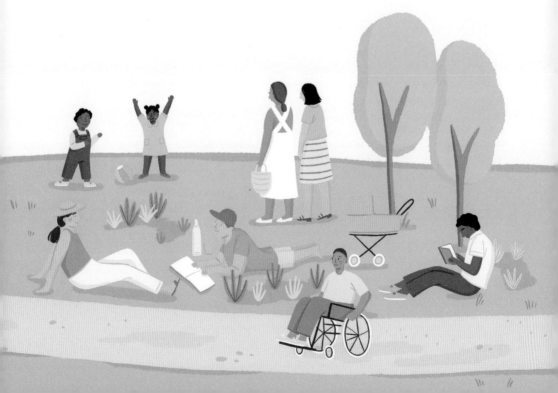

TRY THIS...

Some Tips for Sunday-ing

Even with the best of intentions to let go and relax at the weekends, many of us find we inadvertently get caught up in chores and busy work that mean we are just as fatigued by the end of the weekend as we were when it began – sometimes more so. For this reason, the art of Sunday-ing is one to be taken seriously and not left to chance. Sure, we all have obligations – weekday or weekend – but when we put appropriate boundaries around our relaxation time, however little of this time we have available to us, it is much more likely to happen. Try these tips for planning a slow Sunday and recharge in the spirit of *domingueando*.

Make the time

Even if you have commitments that mean a lazy Sunday of sleeping until 10am and having nothing more on the agenda than a relaxed brunch is unlikely to say the least, there is usually at least a pocket of time on a Sunday that can be dedicated to life in the slow lane. From two hours to twenty minutes, whatever time you have, be sure to demarcate it fiercely for *domingueando*.

Make it intentional

Whatever time you have for *domingueando*, approach it with purpose. While slumping in front of the television may feel like all you want to do, this is not always very restorative and can simply keep us in a perpetuated state of lethargy. Instead, try a gentle walk, some slow exercise, a long bath, reading a book or another focussed activity that is both restful and recuperative. You will feel the benefits of *domingueando* far more this way.

Make it mutual

If you have a partner or children, the best way to ensure dedicated *domingueando* time is to involve everyone. This also offers a sense of accountability. When we express to others that we want to incorporate dedicated slowing down time into our week, it is far more likely that we will make this happen. If you live alone, get this accountability by sharing your plans with a friend (like a gym or running partner, but a slowing-down partner!).

Make it a habit

Now that you have your time slot, intentional relaxation ritual and you have made yourself accountable to others by sharing your Sunday activity, all that is left is to be sure that this ritual sticks. Set a recurring alert on your phone – and use this as a prompt to *switch off* your phone for the duration of time you have for *domingueando*. This way you will be reminded every week to enjoy your own little slice of Sunday slowness.

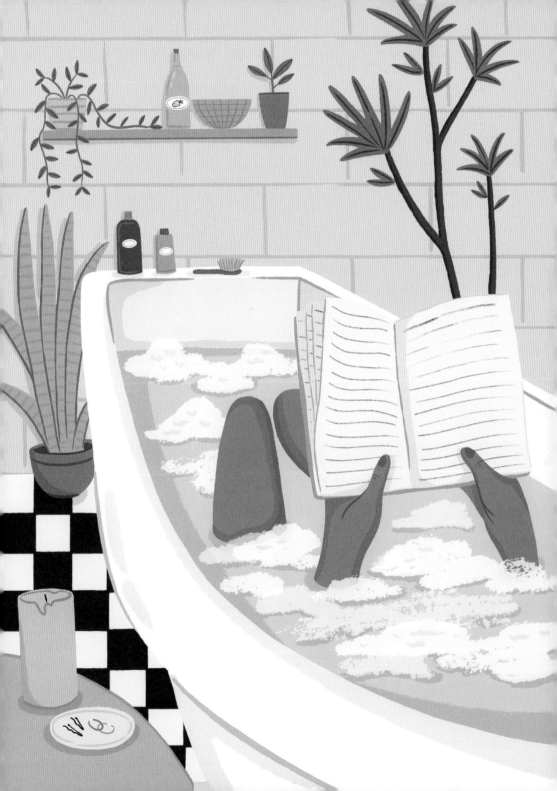

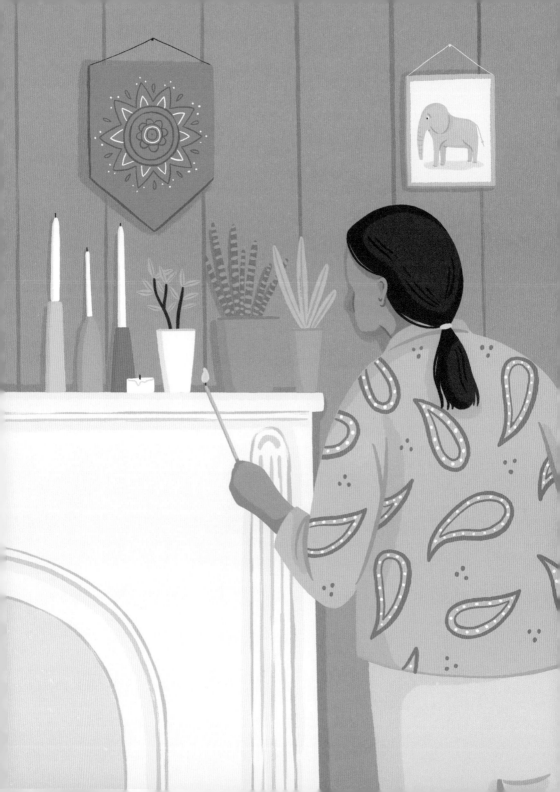

SADHANA

'sɑːðənɑː | noun | Indian
1. dedicated practice or learning

There are many ways in which we might go about making calm a habit in our lives. What lies behind any such committed ritual, however, is the spirit in which we commit. Sometimes it matters less what we pledge to do in order to keep calm, and more how steadfast we are in keeping up such a habit. Enter the Indian concept of *sadhana*, meaning a dedicated practice that furthers one along their spiritual path.

This term comes from the Sanskrit *sādhanā*, meaning 'dedication to an aim' and also from *sādh*, which means to 'bring about'. This concept is not about performing any specific practice per se, but captures the very spirit of keeping up a practice at all – emphasising how beneficial even the simplest ritual can be when it is performed regularly and with dedication.

While creating a *sadhana* might seem easy enough, we will all have had experiences of trying to establish certain habits and then repeatedly letting this slip off our schedules. Therefore, if you want to establish a new *sadhana* of calm in your life, rather than setting yourself a grandiose goal such as thirty minutes of harmonious yoga or meditation each morning at dawn, it might be advisable to start with something a whole lot smaller.

Creating and committing to a small *sadhana* – something as simple, perhaps, as lighting a single candle at the same time every day – may seem somewhat trivial. Yet, like anything, it is the intention we channel into this activity that makes it significant and meaningful in our lives. If your small *sadhana* is to light a candle, you can choose to instil this action with a certain calming intention that holds meaning for you, perhaps encapsulated within a particular word or phrase that you can say aloud, or simply keep in your mind. You may like to make this calming intention an aspirational one, using the action to focus on a certain goal or value that you hold dear. In this way, every time you practise your *sadhana* you will remember something foundational about the person you are. This will help you to reconnect with and remember a subtle, interior sense of your selfhood – something that can be otherwise forgotten in the chaos of daily life.

TRY THIS...

Create a Simple Morning *Sadhana*

You may have found that when you attempt to establish a new habit, all of a sudden, and with alarming consistency, a cascade of reasons *not* to keep it up rush to mind. You might say to yourself that you are too busy, that you are too tired, that there is not enough time, that the habit is self-indulgent, that you do not feel like it, that you will get to it later (knowing you will not get to it later), that you would rather do something else instead... and so on. The best way to beat this tendency is to start small: the smaller the *sadhana*, the less likely your multitude of excuses will be to hold water. Not only this, but your success with a small *sadhana* may just spur you onward in extending your practice further. Here are some ideas for beginning:

Keep your *sadhana* simple

The simpler your first *sadhana*, the better. Even if you intend to extend your practice further, begin with just the bare essentials. This might mean simply sitting on your yoga mat for one minute. Later you can add further steps to your *sadhana*, and you may also find that – once you sit on the mat for that one minute – you *want* to do some additional stretching, meditation, focused breathing or journal writing... but your *sadhana* need only be that one minute of sitting. Completing this – and only this – every single day will be your success.

Gather the essentials

If your simple *sadhana* involves sitting on your yoga mat, make this experience as

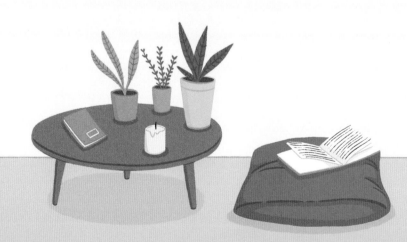

pleasurable as possible. You may like to incorporate a warm shawl to wrap around your shoulders, a soft cushion to sit on, a small candle to light and possibly a journal to capture your first thoughts of the day. Gather the items and objects that will make this practice feel relaxing and enjoyable for you. The better your *sadhana* feels, the easier it will be to keep up.

Practise your *sadhana* first thing in the morning
Have everything you need in place, perhaps set up in a corner of your bedroom, so that you can go straight from your bed to your *sadhana* with the fewest obstacles possible. The good thing about this is that you will start every day with a sense of triumph if you complete your *sadhana*.

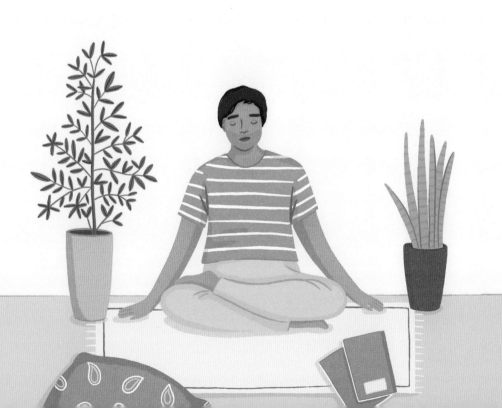

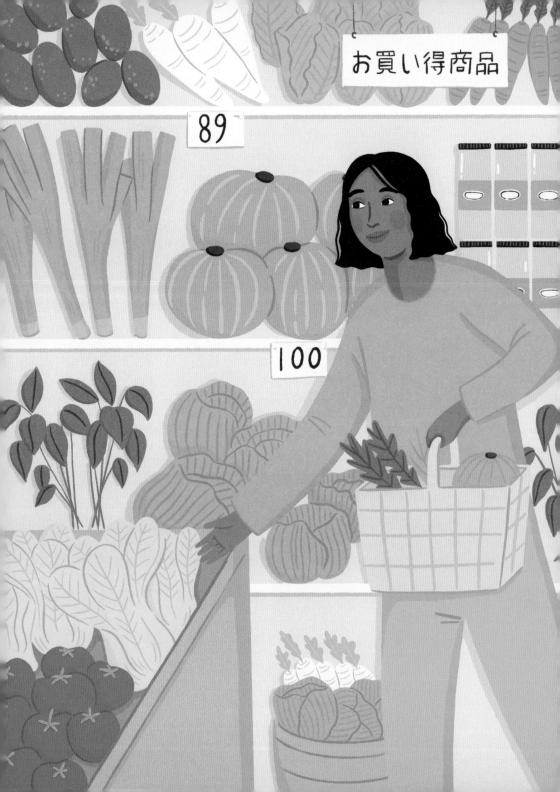

NUCHI GUSUI

ŋuːʃiːɡuːʃiː | Proverb | Japanese (from Okinawa)
1. to treat one's food as medicine for living

Around the world we engage in the ritual of eating in incredibly varied ways – some more conducive to our wellbeing than others. The typical 'Western' diet includes some particularly bad habits, such as high consumption of red meat and low consumption of fruit and vegetables. At the opposite end of the scale there is one particular place in the world that has been revered for its eating habits (and particularly how conducive these are to a long and healthy life): the Japanese island of Okinawa.

In this unique place, food is not simply a source of energy or pleasure. Food, for Okinawans is ritualistically revered as remedial and life-sustaining. The diet in Okinawa has traditionally included vegetables as a staple, plenty of soy protein and a limited amount of lean meat and seafood. This concept is captured by the Okinawan proverb *nuchi gusui*, or 'food is medicine'. It is this special reverence for food that also appears to inform the Okinawan habit of *hara hachi bu*, or eating until you are only 'eight parts full' for health and longevity. This traditional way of approaching mealtimes has an increasingly sound basis in contemporary science: sensible calorie restriction has shown to have positive health effects in studies on eating habits.

These two key habitual differences – both of revering what our food does for us and also practising a *less is more* habit of how we consume food – certainly seem to have done the Okinawan people multiple favours. These people are recognised around the world for their longevity. Okinawa is considered a 'blue zone', one of the places where people live longer than anywhere else. Is it time that we all made the ritual of eating a little more sacred, and a little less swift?

TRY THIS...

Eat the *Nuchi Gusui* Way

Eating can be calm and mindful, or it can be a rushed affair where we guzzle down our food at great speed so that we can get back to work as soon as possible (as it has increasingly become in the West). We all *have* to eat, but sometimes it is *how* we eat that makes all the difference. Mealtimes offer us the opportunity to practise ritualistically slowing down to revere and respect our food. If you would like to make eating a little calmer and more conducive to health, have a go at these ideas to help you adopt the habit of *nuchi gusui*.

Start with simple healthy habits

Getting into the habit of treating your food as medicinal does not mean waiting until you are ill and hoping to cure your fever with a bowl of green vegetables. Rather, it is recognising that every meal is an opportunity to stockpile key vitamins and minerals that will *keep* you well. You might like to start small, by adding some ground flaxseed to your porridge (rich in Omega-3), swapping to multigrain bread from white, adding extra immune-boosting garlic to meals that you already like to cook or taking a good-quality multivitamin supplement. Once you have introduced these smaller habits, bigger changes such as upping your vegetable intake and cutting back on red meat will likely feel easier.

Make your plate a rainbow

Once you have habitualised the small changes above and started to treat mealtimes as an opportunity for a ritualistic health boost and not merely a way to gratify a growling tummy, you might like to step things up a notch. The Okinawan diet revolves around plant foods – and yours can too! Wave farewell to five-a-day and strive for ten portions of fruit and vegetables a day. A simple and easy way to know you are getting the greatest range of health benefits from the plants you eat is this: aim for a variety of colours. Orange sweet potato and carrots, red peppers, yellow peppers, green leafy vegetables, purple cabbage, white onions... the broader the range of colours on your plate, the greater the range of vitamins and minerals you will be getting. Simple.

Take your time and drink more water

As well as making healthier eating choices, we must also think about how we help ourselves to digest these foods so as to avoid leaving our bodies operating at a disadvantage. We need to be well hydrated in order to effectively digest our food and extract the nutrients it contains, so be sure to have a large glass of water around half an hour before every meal. Try also giving yourself ten minutes extra to eat each meal: chew slower, take a moment between mouthfuls and try to notice when you become full rather than overeating as a result of being on autopilot.

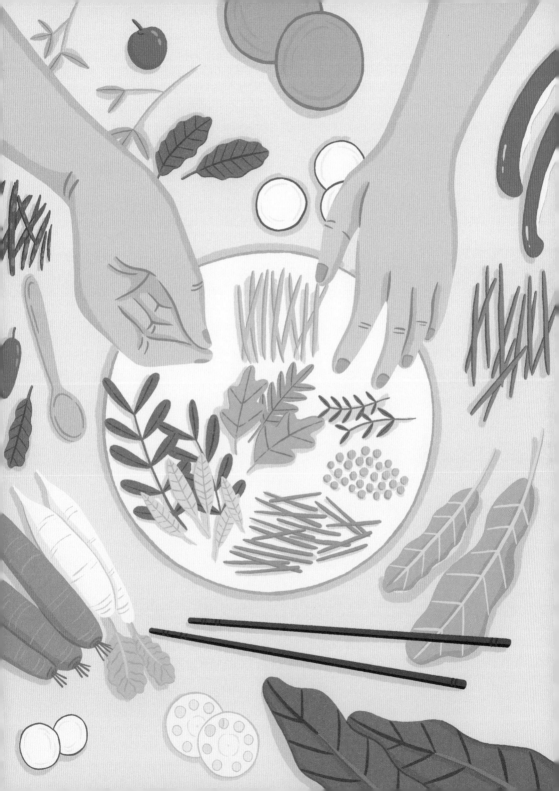

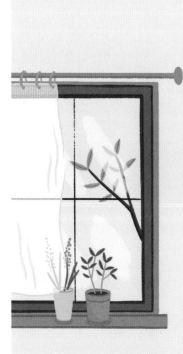

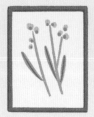

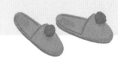

CHAPTER FOUR

Rest & Relaxation

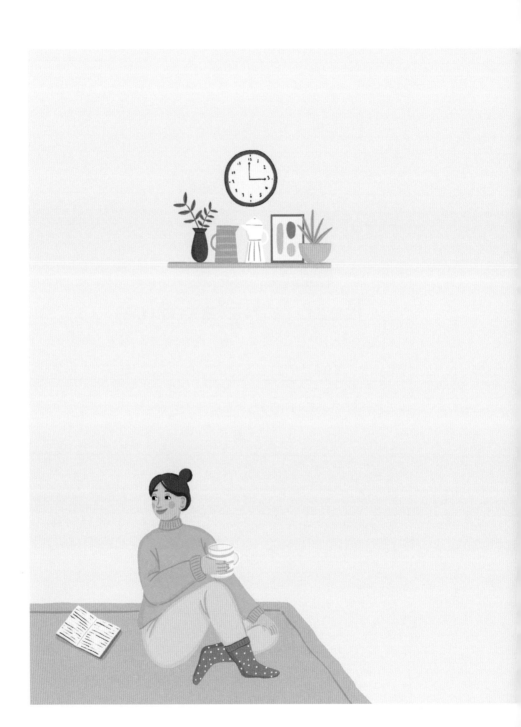

While there will always be new-fangled trends around how we can keep our minds and bodies calm, it is hard to beat that most straightforward and time-honoured way of practising serenity: simply putting our feet up and having a rest. Relaxing in a cosy seat, dozing, napping, lounging and getting enough sleep are perhaps some of the most valuable forms of self-care there are, and are well-practised habits we all share. We all know what it feels like to kick back in hammocks, switch off accidentally on public transport, nod off in our armchairs and cuddle up for quick kips with those we love. We even endorse 'sleeping on it' when things are troubling us, because we know that taking time to rest is essential to seeing clearly and feeling good.

Yet even the peaceful pastime of simple rest has manifested itself in unique ways around the world, epitomised through certain words and practices that highlight exactly how our different cultures like to get their forty winks, or simply get some downtime (*lying down* time, that is). Across the world we have found terms that evoke sleepiness after meals, dozing off in the heat and the bright feeling of mornings when we have slept particularly well.

We all treasure the feeling of being well rested, and also know how easy it is to become burnt out when we fail to prioritise relaxation. We are all guilty of pouring ourselves into work and commitments that result in us feeling weary rather than reposed. Take the time now (or perhaps in those quiet moments before bed) to peruse this chapter and consider some different interpretations of a globally cherished pastime: rest and relaxation. They might just help you to think differently about how you restore and revive yourself.

FREDAGSMYS

freɪndæsmiːs | compound noun | Swedish
1. Friday cosiness

At times, the pressure to use our weekends for extravagant bouts of
socialising can feel like having a second full-time job. There we are,
exhausted from our commutes, tired out from juggling our to-do lists
and weary from suffering endless work meetings. Somehow, in this
bedraggled state, we are then expected to throw on our glad rags and
get out on the town come Friday. Where, oh where, is the time for simply
taking it easy and not doing much at all? And, more importantly, how do
we celebrate this as an intentional and pleasurable activity in-and-of itself
and not simply a fatigued retreat from the hubbub of daily reality, laced
with a sense of 'FOMO', or a 'fear of missing out'? The Swedish people
have the perfect solution and they call it *Fredagsmys*.

This term is formed by compounding *Fredag*, which means 'Friday',
with *mys*, which means 'cosiness', and is a pursuit that is treasured in
Swedish culture: staying home on a Friday evening to share easy-to-

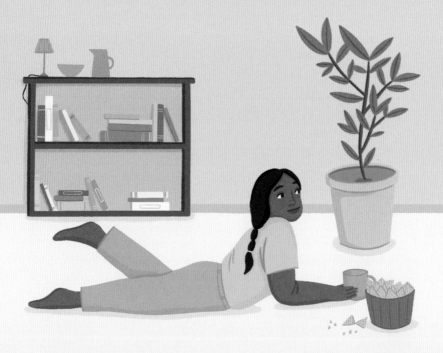

prepare food with loved ones, while watching television and snuggling together on the sofa. You might also come across this concept in verb form, *fredagsmysa* (to have a cosy Friday night in) – you could ask a friend, 'shall we *fredagsmysa* tonight?'.

This concept reportedly arose colloquially some time in the mid 1990s, before gaining pride of place in the Swedish dictionary, and it is now a beloved pastime shared by Swedes from all walks of life. Whoever you are and whatever you do, after a long week you will still be likely to appreciate the special treat of *Fredagsmys*.

Indeed, in Sweden, *mys* is such a serious business that there are all manner of specific forms of getting cosy. You might hear *höstmys* or 'autumn cosiness', which captures that special sensation of layering up and staying indoors as the air turns crisp and cool following a hot summer. There is also the specific delight of *julmys* or 'Christmas cosiness', and the more general *kvällsmys* or 'evening cosiness'. Of these, however, *Fredagsmys* is the term you will likely hear the most often, and is a practice that has become something of a nationally cherished custom. Did you need more of an excuse to simply stay home at the end of a long week and celebrate all things cosy? Well, now you have it.

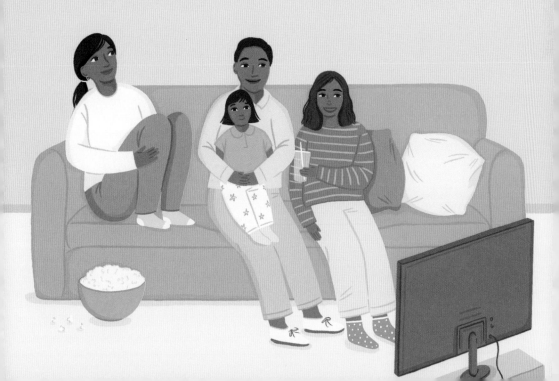

TRY THIS...

Schedule a Night of *Fredagsmys*

If you have found that the pressure to be a party animal once the weekend arrives has gradually become less and less appealing, then *Fredagsmys* may be the ideal antidote. Scheduling a night of Friday cosiness is the perfect pastime to introduce to your end-of-the-week agenda when you are feeling world-weary. Luckily, and rather aptly, it requires little more than grabbing a few blankets and snacks and settling down in front of the television with those you love. Follow these tips to create your own cosy Friday night in, the Swedish way.

1. The first main requirement to ensure you are doing *Fredagsmys* right, lies in creating a *mysig* environment. This word implies a broad sense of contentment and evokes anything that affords us a feeling of comfort and warmth. A *mysig* atmosphere can therefore easily be created with low lighting, candles, cushions and blankets for that extra element of cosiness. The idea is to create a sacred space where you can snuggle, or *mysa*, in absolute comfort.

2. While one could in theory do *Fredagsmys* by themselves, it is far preferable for Swedes to share these cosy evenings with those they care about – but who this might be is up to you. Everyone can enjoy *Fredagsmys* whether they are a family or a group of friends.

3. Oddly enough, one meal that has become synonymous with *Fredagsmys* is the humble taco. This delightful cultural fusion sees the relaxed pace of a Scandinavian evening combined with the ease of a much-loved Mexican delicacy. So, while you might be tempted to simply order a pizza – a completely valid option for an authentic *Fredagsmys* – if you want to make your evening that bit more special and intentional you might consider preparing this simple meal with friends. Gather some delicious ingredients for an easy-to-throw-together feast of fresh and tasty tacos to accompany your evening of staying cosy at home.

4. To sustain your evening of *Fredagsmys* you will likely want some great television to watch. What better viewing material then, than a box set of any one of the brilliantly gritty crime drama series to have emerged from Scandinavia over the years? You will also want to equip yourself with a range of salty and sweet snacks including crisps, popcorn and candy to nibble on as your Friday night unfolds in blissful repose.

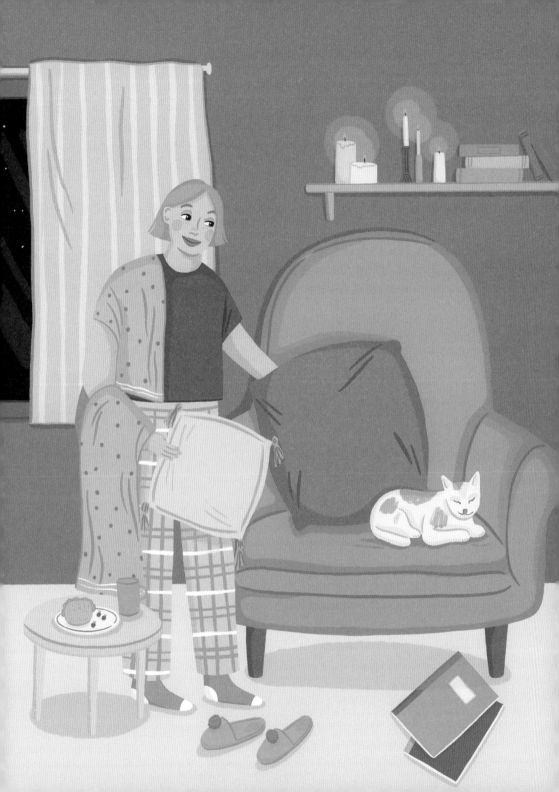

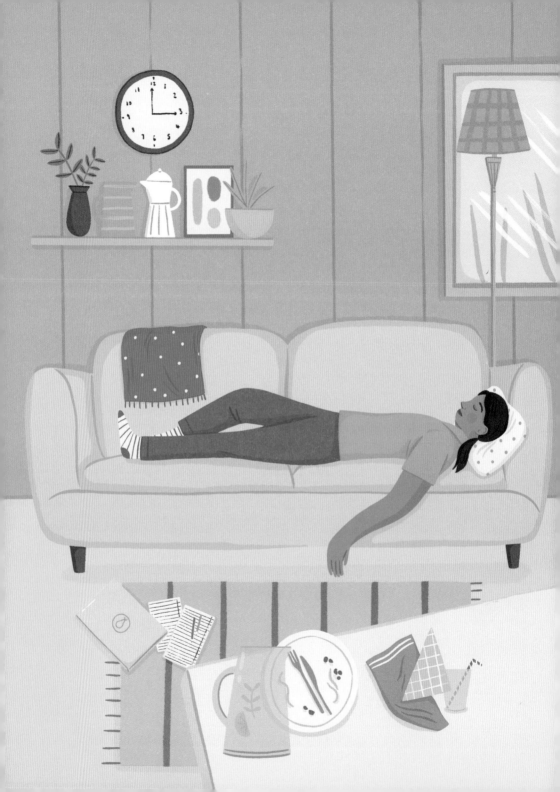

ABBIOCCO

ab'bjɔkko | noun | Italian
1. drowsiness, particularly after a large meal

Whatever our age or walk of life – from babies and young children to mid-life and older age – all of us can appreciate the joys of a good nap. While most of us feel bright and attentive in the first part of the day, we will all know the phenomenon of post-lunch lethargy. It seems fitting, then, that the culture that has found a word to precisely capture this feeling is a culture that does lunch with particular aplomb: Italy. After several courses of rich and delicious sauce-covered carbohydrates, even the best of us would benefit from forty winks – and it is exactly this feeling that is evoked by *abbiocco*. This word translates simply as 'drowsiness' or to 'surrender to fatigue' but in common usage often relates to the particular kind of fatigue that results from a full stomach – an experience that the Italian people know all too well as some of the world's biggest food lovers (and no strangers to hearty meals). As food is such an important part of any given day in this country, you may be likely to hear something along the lines of *dopo pranzo mi viene l'abbiocco*, or 'after lunch I always get drowsy'.

Of course, you do not have to find yourself in this nation of pasta pioneers to experience the warm, sleepy feeling that often follows eating. Perhaps you had the best of intentions to enjoy a night out dancing, but after dinner found your resolve quashed. Or maybe at the office you saved a big bit of work for after lunch only to find yourself falling asleep at your desk and unable to concentrate. When our digestion is working double time then the rest of us, well, it does not want to work at all. The solution? Embrace the Italian feeling of *abbiocco* and let yourself rest while you digest. If you are at home, take a quick nap. If you are at work, ensure you avoid leaving tough tasks until after lunch and stick to simpler admin tasks instead. Or (if all else fails) you could always counter *abbiocco* with an equally Italian *espresso*.

FJAKA

/fjâka/ | noun | Croatian
1. sleepiness; relaxation of body and mind; doing nothing; daydreaming

While the cooler climes of the world have developed many ways of describing the cosy comfort of hiding indoors and escaping cold weather, our warmer countries and continents have crafted a range of ways to conjure up quite the opposite feeling: relaxing in the heat of the sun. When it is particularly warm there is often nothing for it but to succumb to slowing down and taking a load off. Intense heat means that rest becomes obligatory, and all else must wait. It is this spirit that is captured by the Croatian term *fjaka*.

   Fjaka is another of those curiously untranslatable words that cannot quite be captured in specific detail outside of its original environs. Yet we can probably all get a sense of what it attempts to capture:

that day-dreamy, drowsy state that excessive heat can induce, where work is the farthest thing from our minds. At these times, we enter into an absent-minded, almost meditative, state.

When experiencing *fjaka*, Croatians may succumb to drowsiness, to the detriment of any prior engagements – but there is really nothing else for it. When the heat swells, *fjaka* will not be far behind. You may even hear the phrase 'alas, my friends, *fjaka* has caught me!'. What better way to say 'no' to the constant demands of the world?

Perhaps you have fallen into *fjaka* only rarely – maybe when you were on a sunny holiday overseas, or during summer months relaxing in the garden or on a walking weekend by the coast. Perhaps, if you hail from a hot country, *fjaka* might be something you encounter on a daily basis. It could be that you must build your life around *fjaka*, by waking early to be productive in the cooler morning hours for instance, so that the hot afternoons can be reserved for rest.

It can be challenging for some us to embrace the unproductivity inherent to *fjaka*. Yet we can opt to see rest as productive too. As we all know – everything works better when you switch it off and on again.

TRY THIS...

Embrace *Fjaka* with a 'Not-to-do' List

We all have a remarkable talent for filling our time; with work, day-to-day chores, caring for others, striving towards personal goals, trying to get through that stack of books we have been meaning to read... the list goes on. Oh, how the list goes on – quite literally. A great many of us write daily to-do lists as a force of habit. We scribble away our days in a frenzy of efficiency. In fact, with the recent trend towards bullet journalling, the once humble to-do list has become something of a cult-craze.

When did our days and weeks cease to feel like precious time that we should savour, and instead become a series of commoditised units of potential productivity? It is unclear precisely when we collectively agreed to live our lives in this way, but all this wringing out of the time available to us in life is making us feel, well, rather wrung out ourselves.

Yet, a more tranquil existence is within our grasp, if we wish to opt for it. We can all choose to reclaim – in both large and small ways – our rest time. We can champion our identity as a human *being* (as opposed to a human *doing*), and we can prioritise our peacefulness. What is more is that we will not be alone if we do, and we can take heart from this fact. As *fjaka* and the other wonderfully calming terms in this book show, many cultures around the world actively bypass the wrung-out way of life. They do this by privileging unproductivity, celebrating distraction and reveling in reverie – and you can, too.

While it may at first feel remarkably uncomfortable to simply... stop doing so much, it seems to increasingly be the life goal *du jour*. We just aren't sure how we can possibly get away with it. Today, not doing all that much has become a highly privileged position – such that it feels as though the only way to achieve a state of non-doing is to do *even more* right now to help us get there (wherever 'there' might be for us: the fabled state of liberated self-employment, retirement, etc.). Yet the illogicality of this is self-evident. Somewhere in our hearts we already recognise ourselves as the proverbial rats on the racing wheel.

Choose to counter this trend in the simplest way: if you insist on a to-do list (we all know they are necessary at times), compliment this with a not-to-do list, too. What gets written on there is up to you – the key is simply realising what can wait. What can you get away with not doing today? Cast it off in the spirit of *fjaka*. When this becomes your habit – rather than relentlessly filling your days to the brim – life might just start to feel a little more restful, exactly as it is.

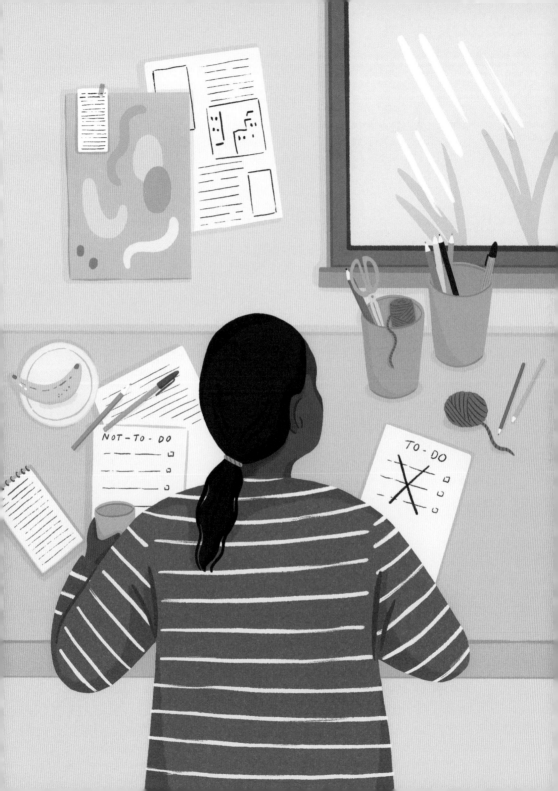

THE SERENITY
OF SLUMBER

As babies we all nap regularly, and this is recognised as an essential part of our early brain development. Yet it is not just at this early stage when sleep has a profound impact upon our health and wellbeing, and it is not only our brains that benefit when we snooze. As adults, not only does sleep help us feel calm and rested but, in our hours of slumber, almost every tissue in our body is working hard at repairing and restoring itself. Sleep affects our immune systems, our blood pressure, our appetite and even our cardiovascular health.

To gain the greatest of restorative benefits, experts say, it is vital that adults get between seven to eight hours of sleep per night. This allows for the optimum 'good night' of four to five sleep cycles. In each cycle, we progressively enter states of deep sleep and rapid eye movement (REM) sleep – the kind of sleep in which we dream.

Unfortunately, many aspects of modern life intrude upon and disrupt us from getting the best night of slumber possible, including too much caffeine, certain medications and electronic light from our gadgets. Yet in cultures around the world, even if sleep is missed in the nighttime hours, a daytime snooze is perfectly acceptable – if not actively encouraged.

The Japanese have refined the art of *inemuri* (居眠り), or the practice of dozing in public. This might be on public transport, or even at one's desk – and it is often seen as a sign of hard work to productively nap in this way (understandably, given that lack of sleep impairs concentration).

In the Mediterranean, the tradition of the nap is a longstanding one. Most of us have heard of the Spanish *siesta*, a time where small shops and business will often close so that locals can escape the heat to snooze. The Italians call this afternoon retreat *riposo*, or *meriggiare* (to rest at noon in the shade).

From India we find 'yogic sleep' or yoga *nidra* (योग निद्रा), which describes the deliberate practice of entering the state just between sleep and fully wakeful consciousness, in order to deeply relax.

Finally, who says we need to retreat to our beds alone, at night or at naptime? The Dutch recognise the serene art of *kweesten*, or the act of 'chatting in bed with one's lover'.

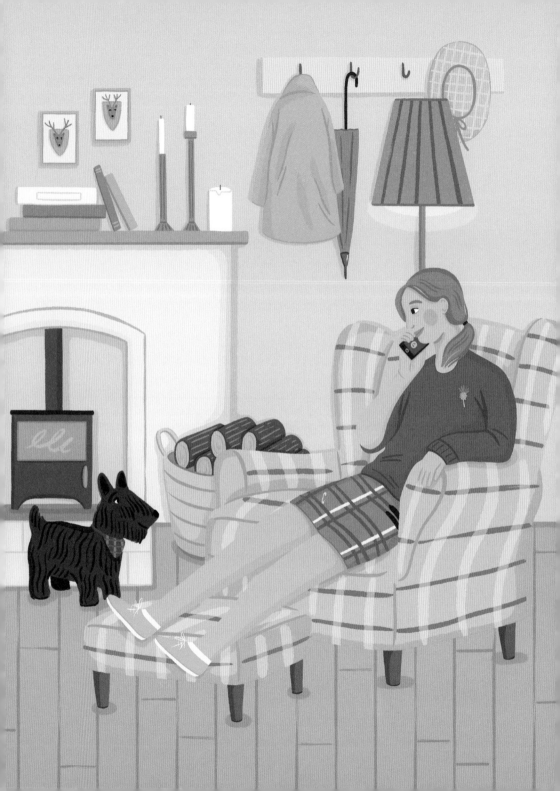

COUTHIE

ˈkuθi | adjective | Scottish
1. (of a person) amiable, friendly, sympathetic
2. (of a thing or place) comfortable, snug

Both physical places and particular people evoke all manner of relaxed and restful feelings in us. Having someone we love and care for around us can make us feel as equally 'at home' as we would if we were literally at home. Equally, an uncomfortable or unpleasant environment can be made infinitely better by having someone there with us who evokes feelings of comfort and pleasantness. Sometimes it is the restful and relaxed company of another person that will help us to feel the most serene – rather than escaping to some remote island to get away from it all.

The lovely Scottish term of endearment, *couthie*, appears to capture this concept beautifully. *Couthie* can be used to describe both a comfortable or snug physical space and a friendly or amiable person. Originating from the Middle English word *couth*, meaning 'familiar', *couthie* highlights how both familiar places and people draw out similar emotional responses in us. In other words, we feel as safe and relaxed in the presence of certain special others as we do in snug and tranquil spaces. Both evoke a feeling of being supported and safe, free to unwind and help us to switch out of high alert and sit our world-weary selves down for a while. *Couthie*, then, seems quintessentially Scottish in its cosy familiarity; after all, Scotland is a place of warming whisky, welcoming people and comfy tartan furnishings!

All of us find a sense of safety in the familiar. We return to situations where we can rest peacefully among what we know, free from surprise or uncertainty. Consciously comforting ourselves with familiar *couthie* environments and friends could never be one-size-fits-all, but we could certainly all do with more of it. Whatever feels most *couthie* to you – a chat on the phone with a kindly friend, or a snug living room lit by candles where you can rest with a good book – add a dose of that to your day, and unwind in the comfort of the familiar.

MORGENFRISK

ˈmɒɒnˌfʁæsɡ | adjective | Danish
1. morning freshness; feeling rested when you wake up in the morning

There are few better feelings than waking up after a night of deep and rejuvenating sleep, with sunlight peeping through the curtains, stretching your arms above your head and hopping out of bed full of energy for the day. If it were possible to bottle this feeling and put a label on it, the Danish would opt for *morgenfrisk* – a word that evokes the freshness one feels upon waking.

For Danes, the opposite of *morgenfrisk* is *morgensur*, or to be very grumpy first thing in the morning – a feeling with which many of us will be familiar. Yet most Danes would likely fall into the former category, because Denmark is oft regarded as one of the happiest nations in the world; this is a country of optimists that make a habit of seizing the day.

Whether you tend towards *morgenfrisk* or *morgensur*, there are little things we can all do to experience brighter mornings – not least by getting an earlier night. It is a worthwhile investment to get those extra hours of snooze time because feeling fresh and alert in the morning can make all the difference to the day ahead. In Danish schools, teachers might ask the children in their classes, *er du frisk?* or 'are you fresh?'. We all know that an alert and lively mind is best for learning, but even when our school days are behind us we can benefit in all kinds of ways from feeling *morgenfrisk*. A feeling of freshness in the morning can help us to be more productive throughout the day, to make better and more focused decisions and to be less snappy with others – highlighting the importance of a relaxed and restful night's sleep, whatever age we are.

Not all of us find sleep straightforward, and this means that not all of us get the bright *morgenfrisk* mornings we deserve. In the modern world, our days are inundated with emails and texts and demands and pings and prods and bleeps and endless alerts so that, when we come to switch off at night, we can find that it is impossible to unplug and unwind. Try avoiding technology for the last hour, or even two hours, of your day – opting for reading, stretching or writing in a journal as a more calming way to end your day, and wake up feeling a little more *morgenfrisk*.

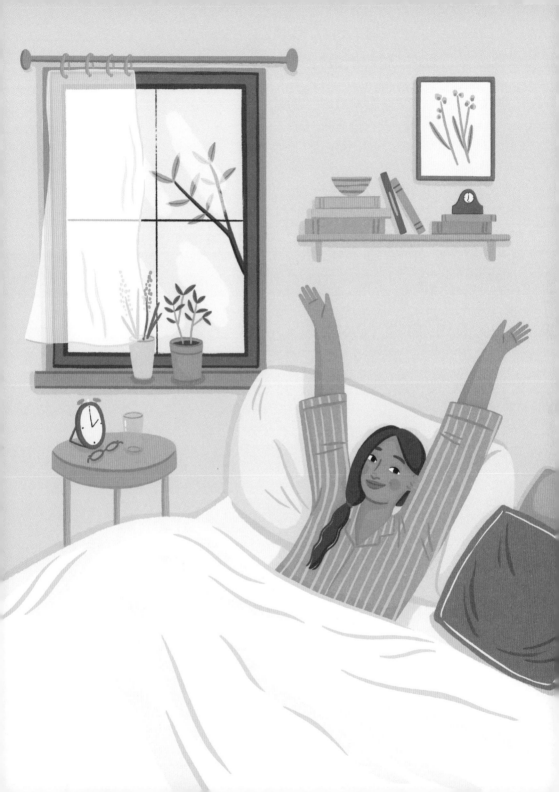

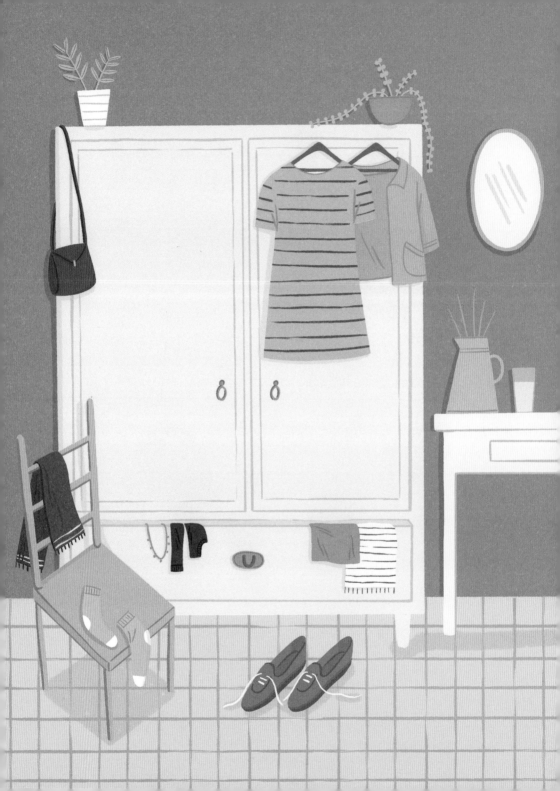

TRY THIS...

Make Your Morning More *Morgenfrisk*

If there is one secret to an energised morning, it is a relaxed and tranquil night of sleep. Yet even after a night that is more rest*less* than *restful*, there are simple, stimulating morning rituals that can help the early hours feel a little less frazzled and a little more *morgenfrisk*.

Three tips for a more *morgenfrisk* morning:

1. **Drink a glass of water.** Most of us turn to caffeine first thing to put a little pep in our step. While there is nothing necessarily wrong with this, even the most die-hard coffee lovers among us require more rehydration than a latte or cappuccino are ever going to provide. When you pop the kettle on for your first cuppa, add a little extra water in to boil. When boiled, top up half a glass of cold water with some hot and drink this down before your tea or coffee. You will find that slightly warm water is much easier to drink than cold, and this simple habit will help hydrate you after a long night.

2. **Wake up and smell the... lavender?** Our sense of smell is powerful and scents like lavender can not only relax us but also put us in a better mood (as well as help us to maintain a good mood). In a study where lavender oil burners were introduced to a workplace environment over a 3-month period, almost 90% of respondents from a total of 66 individuals felt more positive about the environment. Invest in an oil burner and light it first thing when you wake up to get a good mood boost from the get-go. Alternatively, you could also look out for shower products with lavender oil.

3. **Dress without stress.** There are few things more frustrating than getting ready for work in the morning and finding nothing clean to wear. Yet feeling good in what we are wearing – and getting dressed calmly, as opposed to in a sweaty and flustered panic – is an easy way to capture the essence of *morgenfrisk*. Before going to sleep, get in the habit of setting out what you will wear the next day. This simple habit will soon become routine and save you many a *morgensur* morning.

VILLASUKKAPÄIVÄ

viːlæsuːkəpaɪdə | compound noun | Finnish
1. a woollen socks day

Picture the scene: you are reclining on a comfortable sofa, white snow is glistening outside the window of your country log cabin, a fire is crackling in the grate, you have no particular plans for the day, nothing to stress you out, and there is steam gently rising from the hot drink at your elbow that is just waiting to be sipped in total and complete tranquillity.

Within this peaceful visualisation, I challenge you to look down at your imaginary feet and to not see a pair of thick woollen socks. Somehow, woollen socks are the only appropriate footwear for this country cabin day of retreat. The Finnish people know this, and have thus duly captured the entire scenario outlined above in one perfectly succinct term: *villasukkapäivä*, literally a 'wool sock day'.

For Fins, woollen socks stand for everything that is peaceful, homely, tranquil, warm, safe, traditional and down to earth. For this reason, the word *villasukkapäivä* captures the quiet calm of a day spent with nothing more important on the agenda than to pad around in your woollen socks in total retreat from the outside world.

Taking a *villasukkapäivä* is a chance to wander leisurely around your home (quietly, because of the soft socks), sip warm drinks, read those books that you have been meaning to read, lose yourself in reverie gazing out of the window as the outside world passes by, daydream, gaze out of the window some more and generally press pause on your life. In Finnish culture, this carefree state is summarised and exemplified in a pair of perfectly warm woolly socks – and it is not hard to see why.

If you find yourself feeling that life has got a little too noisy then it might be time to plan your own *villasukkapäivä*. This ceremonious activity of kicking off your outdoor shoes and slipping into a pair of cosy socks might just help you switch modes, slow down and de-stress as you softly amble around your home in complete peace and quiet.

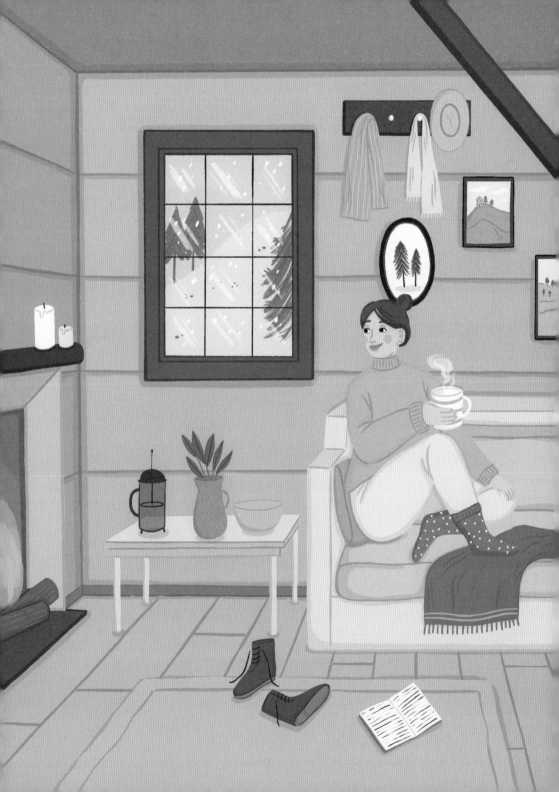

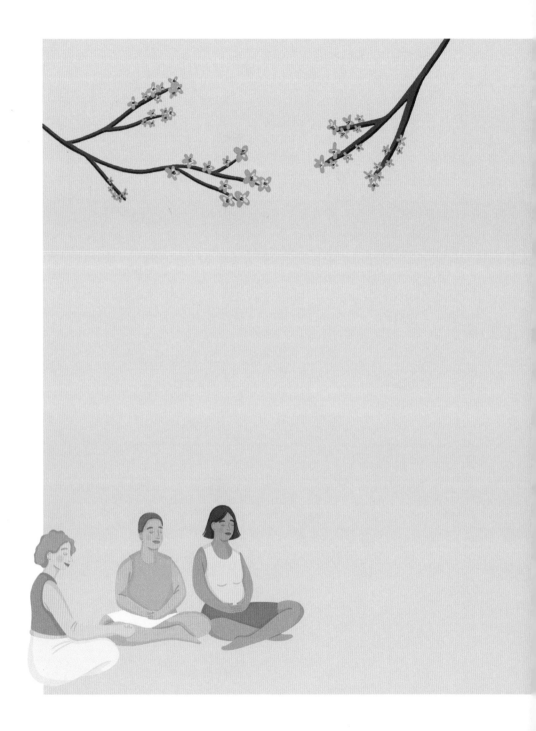

CHAPTER FIVE

Patience & Poise

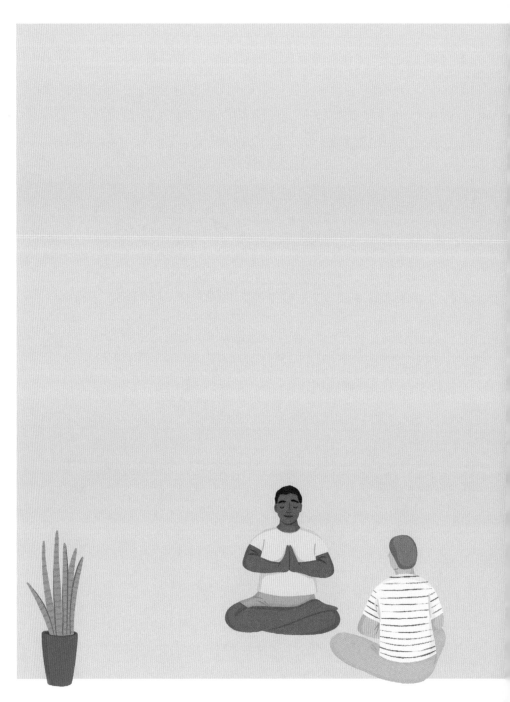

We often seek serenity – not when our jobs are ticking along just fine and our families are being enduringly supportive and our relationships are light and jolly – but at times when quite the opposite is going on. It is when we are faced with the hardest of times – when our patience and poise are critically tested – that we strive most resolutely for serenity. It is on the day that we get told of the redundancies happening at work; or the day that someone we care about is given bad news; or the day that our partner tells us they are unhappy. On these kinds of days, peace of mind can feel a million miles away. Yet, we need only look around us – to our immediate families, communities and to the wider world – to also see how human beings display an astonishing aptitude for resilience during these types of hardships. This resilience is in part thanks to cherished virtues and practices that bolster our resolve.

Of course, maintaining our poise in a crisis is no mean feat. While calm seas make for smooth sailing, when the storm hits we are all liable to veer off course and get lost. We might have the best of intentions before things go wrong, i.e. when times are good – the intention to get along well with and respect other people, for example, or the intention to keep our cool and find a rational solution to any problem. Nevertheless, right there in the thick of disaster, this resolve can waver.

As you navigate the twists and turns of your own life, visit and revisit the words in this chapter. Let them serve as reconciliation and a reminder of the many ways in which we have collectively learned, wherever we are in the world, to sail our way through rough seas, swept onwards by the winds of serenity.

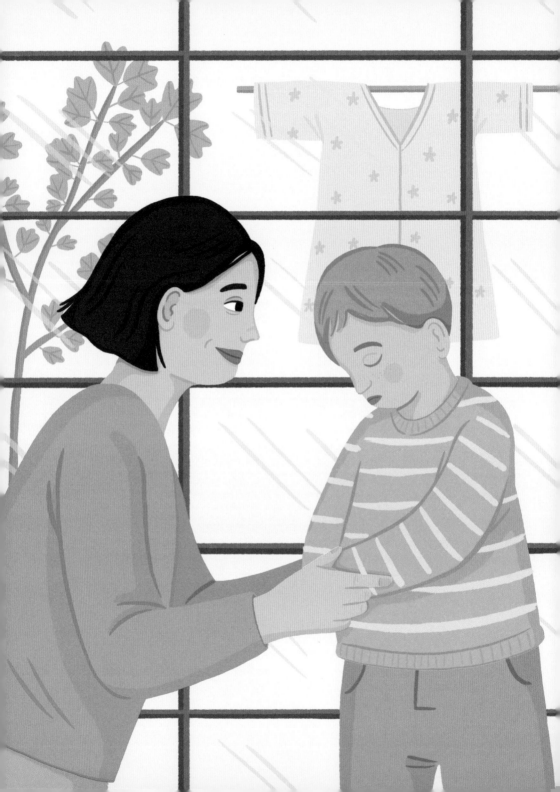

GAMAN (我慢)

/ˈkaːma(ː)n/ | noun and verb | Japanese (from Zen Buddhism)
1. enduring adversity; patience; perseverance; dignity

Feeling serene when our lives are going well is relatively easy. The ability to achieve this state in difficult times – to 'hang in there' – is a good deal harder. This is something that most of us will have experienced at one time or another, and is an idea that is encapsulated in the Japanese concept of *gaman*.

Gaman is a teaching of Zen Buddhism and is a term that evokes a subtle mingling of endurance, patience, dignity and stoic self-discipline. It implies the kind of resolve that prevents us from retaliating to bullies when we know the situation will not be improved by doing so. It is the decision to retreat when necessary because to 'fight back' will only cause us additional distress.

As it endorses quiet perseverance, *gaman* has been associated with passivity in the face of treatment or conditions that one should potentially challenge, rather than endure. However when we consider it a little closer we find that to truly achieve *gaman* is to be far from being passive. Static apathy is not what is implied by this term, but a resolve that requires enormous strength and vigour. It is not always the visible forms of our resistance that count, but the quiet tenacity of interior resistance.

We may not always be able to exercise the strength of *gaman* in difficult times, and we should by no means look at our vulnerability in these times as a weakness. Yet to consider the idea of *gaman* when things are looking tough may just help us to zoom out of seemingly intolerable circumstances and to find a path forwards. In admiring *gaman* in others and in ourselves, we can recognise and revere our collective ability to withstand hardship, to weather the inevitable storms of adversity and to find serenity in even the toughest of circumstances.

TRY THIS...

Bolster your *Gaman* Through Connection

What gives us the determination to go on when we face hardship, as *gaman* promotes? Well, often it is our broader sense of purpose and meaning in life. The late psychoanalyst Viktor Frankl, author of the seminal book, *Man's Search for Meaning*, reportedly used to take his patients by the hand when they first came to him and invite them to join him in jumping out of the window. Whatever came to mind that meant they could not imagine doing such a thing – their partner waiting for them at home, their children, their elderly parents, even a pet they needed to feed – this was where they should start to look for meaning in their life (a risky strategy indeed, and one that would shock any of us into a deep consideration of what really counts).

Few of us spend much time considering the sources of meaning in our lives. It is often only when we are already face-to-face with hardship that we question such things – but it makes little sense to leave such important questions until the point of desperation.

While individual human beings are infinitely diverse, psychologists broadly agree that we find meaning in similar ways. One of the most fundamental of these is our sense of connectedness to others, as is illustrated by the typical responses from Frankl's clients. Explore the following ideas to deepen your own sense of connection with others, and hopefully bolster your ability to practise *gaman*.

Talk it out
There is the age-old saying that a problem shared is a problem halved. We might even go as far as to say that, sometimes, a problem shared is a problem solved. This is because a lack of communication itself can cause us problems. When we stew or ruminate on an issue it can begin to feel increasingly overwhelming. With the perspective of a trusted other, even the most gargantuan of personal struggles can be diminished. Find someone with whom you feel safe opening up, and then make it a regular habit to constructively explore your challenges together.

Get beyond the virtual
Many of us are constantly 'connected' to others through various forms of technology and social media. Yet this rarely results in an authentic sense of connection. Where possible, invest in face-to-face encounters with others as a way to feel supported – beyond the crutch of virtual reality.

Show your gratitude to others
Friends, family and even colleagues often support us in innumerable ways – from the subtle to the more obvious. Whether it is putting the kettle on for us or having our back in an important meeting, we all get help from somewhere and none of us get very far in life without the sustaining influence and support of others. Make sure that you recognise this support when it happens and show your appreciation.

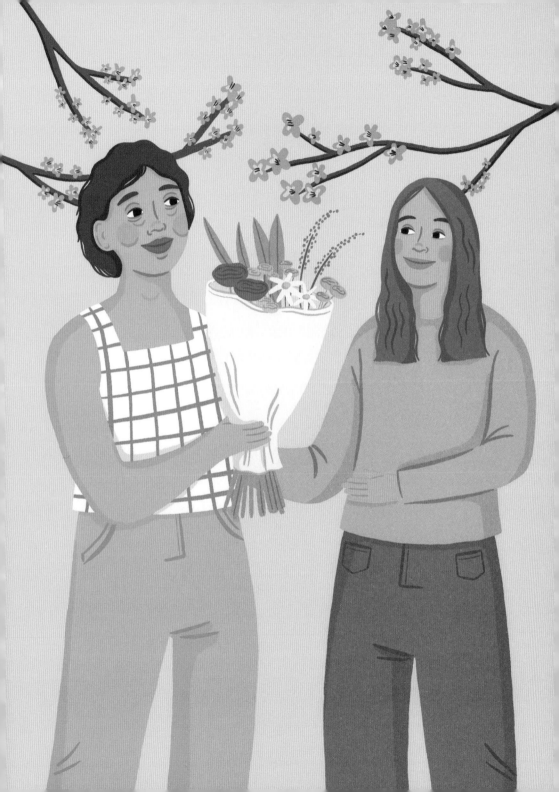

BELUM

/bə.lum/ | verb | Bahasa Indonesia
1. not yet

Uncertainty is, ironically, one of the few certainties of life. Our best-laid plans do not always unfold as we had hoped and, even when they do, we all know that nothing lasts indefinitely. Around the world, therefore, we are united by the fact that each of us will face loss, doubt and times of precariousness. One country that has conceived of a rather unique cultural coping mechanism in the face of this insecurity is Indonesia and their nuanced term *belum*. While this word literally translates as 'not yet', it has a deeper and subtler meaning that implies a calm optimism from which we could all stand to benefit.

    Belum implies possibility without fixating on any outcome in particular. Thus it is inherently humble, reflecting the devoutness of a highly religious country. In this predominantly Muslim nation, *belum* interconnects with the Muslim expression *insha'Allah*, meaning 'God willing'. *Belum* implies hopefulness, while also implying that what one hopes, desires or plans for is – to a degree – out of one's direct control.

Indonesian people can be wary of absolute or definitive statements, and as a rule live far more in the realm of *belum*. This may seem strange until you recognise that this leaves room for even greater possibility and optimism – and, indeed, greater serenity. When we conduct our lives in the spirit of *belum*, joy becomes possible without clinging to certainty, and this is really quite radical to the traditional Western way of thinking. How refreshing to relinquish our misplaced ideas of having jurisdiction over the often quite random and arbitrary ups and downs of life.

In the spirit of *belum*, every positive outcome becomes a gift to which we were never entitled. As a result, we can appreciate it with greater humility. In the spirit of *belum*, every negative outcome can be faced with poise: what we desire may not have happened yet, but there is still time for things to work out better at a later date. Thus, even if we do not consider ourselves to be religious or even spiritual, there is a quietly pragmatic optimism to this term that we could all benefit from adopting.

TRY THIS...

Bye-bye Goals, Hello *Not-Yet* Intentions

Fixating on precise outcomes for our lives is at best naïve and at worst arrogant. While we are typically encouraged in both work life and personal life to calculate specific, measurable goals for what we want, these do not always play out in our favour. This is because life can entail rather more bumps in the road and left-field surprises than we typically reflect upon when listing our goals.

Why not, then, re-conceive of our goals in the light of the *belum* way of thinking? This way, we can allow for much greater fluidity and flexibility in our plans; we exchange arrogance for humility and, as a result, we allow ourselves to pivot when necessary. In letting ourselves be moveable rather than fixed on an ideal, we can then begin to value our general growth and development over conquering any one specific goal or conclusion. Life becomes a series of 'not yets', rather than a desperate grasp for certainties.

Turn to a fresh page in your journal or a notebook and consider the following questions. Hopefully they will serve as a way of crafting some not-yet-realised intentions, rather than rigid goals.

What has not yet happened, but that I hope will happen in my:
  ...career or work life?
  ...creative life/hobbies?
  ...health and fitness?
  ...self-care?

  ...romantic life?
  ...family life?
  ...another domain of life?

Below each of these you may like to note down specific ways that you could act in line with your intentions, in order to see this change come to life. Equally, under each broad question, spend some time reflecting on these further questions:

1. *What are some alternative potential outcomes?*
2. *What if quite the opposite happens – how would that look?*
3. *How will I feel if things do not go the way I hope?*
4. *What might I hope for instead?*
5. *What might an even better outcome of this situation be?*
6. *In what ways will I support myself irrespective of any one particular outcome?*

There is a certain strength and tranquillity that arises when we loosen our grip on getting exactly what we want, lower our expectations and see the positives that can arise from things not going to plan. In fact, when we look back through our past it is often the case that many of the best things that have happened to us, we could never have foreseen or contrived. Plan your life in this spirit, allowing the essence of *belum* to underscore your intentions with gentle humility and (optimistic) detachment from particular outcomes.

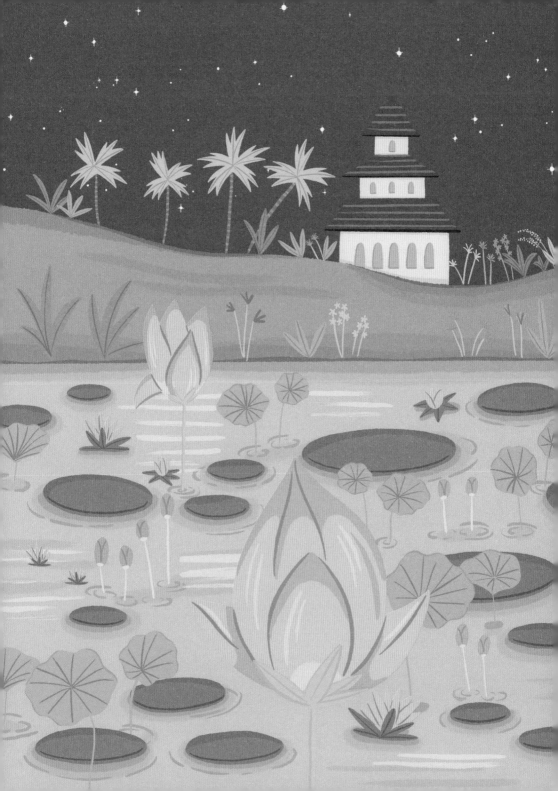

THERE FOR YOU...
FINDING PEACE IN
OTHER PEOPLE

The narrative surrounding serenity can, all across the world, tend towards the solitary. This belief in the need to retreat from the crowd in order to find a bit of peace is, in many ways, understandable. Other people can be unpredictable, loud, brash, intrusive and even offensive at times – perhaps, dare we admit it, one of the greatest sources of our stress. Equally, however (in one of those intense ironies that seem to define all human life on Earth), other people can provide our greatest source of solace. There are many endearing terms across our world's languages that reflect this.

We often find a deep sense of peace and reassurance in the sensation of being part of a collective. The Korean language has a noun for this profound feeling of affection and connectedness between people (that may or may not be romantic): *jeong* (정). Even among Koreans *jeong* is a difficult concept to capture in words. It denotes a kind of shared emotional experience of affinity with another individual or in a group. Somewhat similarly to *jeong* is the Russian noun *sobornost* (собóрность). This term implies a spiritual affinity or unity among jointly living people, which may be religious or secular.

In Urdu, *naz* (ناز) is a word that signifies 'pride', but can be used to more specifically refer to the deeply reassuring confidence in another's love for you being unconditional and steadfast. *Anam ċara:* is a Gaelic expression meaning a 'soul friend', signifying someone that offers you compassionate honesty and a sense of belonging (that is platonic, rather than the specifically romantic English expression, to have a *soul mate*). More romantic is *koi no yokan* (恋の予感), a Japanese phrase that implies a 'premonition of love', or knowing that you will inevitably fall for a person you have just met.

Few – if any – of us are immune to needing others for support and peace of mind. It is through affinity that we feel strong and secure in the face of life's instability. Next time you feel yourself in need of calm and serenity, rather than retreating, why not look to nurture your ties with other people? Instead of meditating alone, consider volunteering your time for a worthy cause in your community, perhaps a homeless shelter or residential home for the elderly. Simply put: when it comes to connectedness, the phrase 'you get what you give' is entirely apt.

UPEKṢĀ (उपेक्षा)

/ʊ.peːk.ʃaː/ | noun | Sanskrit
1. equanimity; a deep state of calm; freedom of mind

We have all experienced what we tend to refer to as the 'ups and downs' of life. We use a range of metaphors for this fluctuating nature of our existence. We lament times when life feels like a 'rollercoaster', or 'the road gets bumpy', 'rocky' or has 'peaks and troughs'. We each face various gains and losses, blessings and calamities, joys and pains, successes and failures – and these sayings figuratively capture our uneasy feelings around such precarious highs and lows.

 At times, we might feel so thrown about by this erraticism that we question how we can ever be expected to maintain our composure in the face of it. Life is just one big lottery, we think, in which we win (and rejoice) or lose (and suffer). Yet, from the Buddhist tradition comes a concept that endorses the development of a sense of freedom from the buffeting nature of our gains and losses: *upekṣā* (or *upekkhā* in Pali). This term evokes a state of profound serenity and composure, no matter what life throws our way. *Upekṣā* is deep inner peacefulness and poise, unaffected by trial or tribulation.

Interestingly, we find a similar idea in the Western philosophical tradition: the ancient Greek concept of *apatheia* (ἀπάθεια). *Apatheia* stems from α- implying 'without' and *pathos* meaning 'passion' or 'suffering'. This should not be confused with the modern-day word 'apathy', which implies a negative indifference. Rather, *apatheia* implies a positive equanimity. The idea is this: with thought and consideration we can cultivate the ability to survive (and thrive) beyond the vacillations of our day-to-day fortunes and misfortunes.

There is a common saying, rooted in stoicism, that decrees how 'pain might be inevitable, but suffering is optional'. It is this idea that seems to underlie both *upekṣā* and *apatheia* – twin concepts that were conjured up in two very distinct corners of the globe, each guiding us towards greater peace of mind amid the mishaps of life.

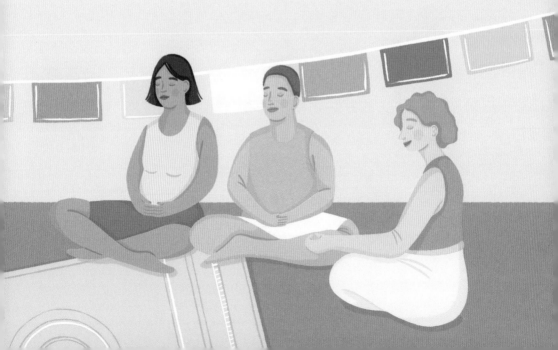

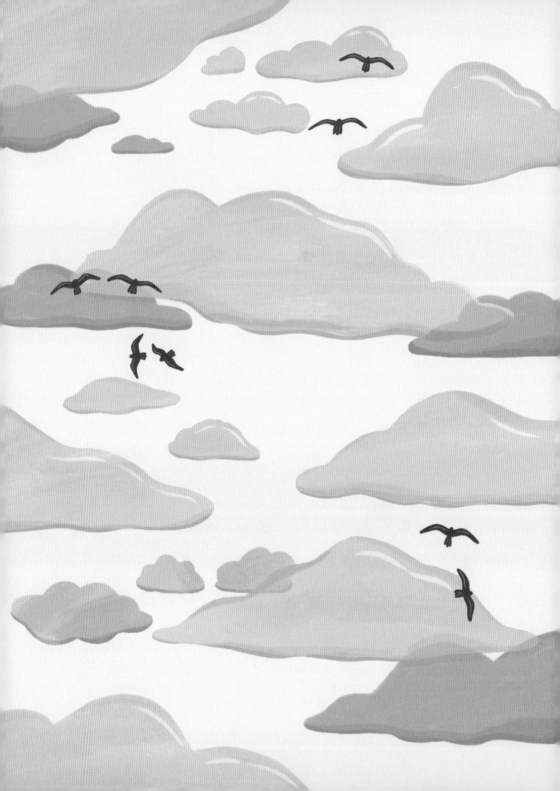

TRY THIS...

Cultivate *Upekṣā* Through Visualisation

Meditation and visualisation are perhaps the best ways to practise *upekṣā*. Through these practices, we can cultivate a sense of distance from external events in a way that is necessary to help us keep our cool. The idea of 'detaching' in this way might feel uncomfortable; for example, if what is bothering us is a cause, person, or group of people we feel passionate about.

Yet it is often only by maintaining this distance that we are able to be of any help at all. Equally, while being concerned about a given issue may be necessary, that does not make it necessary to worry about it constantly – such as when we are trying to sleep at night. If we can cultivate the ability to distance ourselves at certain times, and gift ourselves the necessary break we need from our anxieties, then we equip ourselves to return, renewed, to face them.

Begin by sitting or lying somewhere quiet and comfortable. Gently close your eyes and take several slow, deep breaths. Allow your limbs to soften, and commit to being here in this moment, just as you are.

A short visualisation:
MIND AS SKY, THOUGHTS AS CLOUDS
Try this classic metaphor that brings to light the central aim of meditation. Imagine your mind as an expanse of blue sky. Allow each thought, feeling, sensation, concern, worry or point of anxiety to appear in the sky as a cloud. Some of the clouds might be light and fluffy, while some are heavy and dense. No matter. Allow them all to be there, without judgement. Yet, as you continue to sit quietly and breathe deeply, watch how the clouds gently pass across the sky. Let this illustrate for you how your thoughts and feelings are temporary and fleeting. You are the sky. Your worries pass, and will pass, just as clouds do.

Keep in mind that visualisations tend to be most powerful when related with a personal metaphor that rings true for us. If the above does not strike a chord, think about what might help you particularly to feel distant from life's stressors and achieve a sense of upekṣā – a certain place where you have felt safe and calm, for example – and visualise that in as close detail as possible. You might visualise yourself leaning against a steady oak tree as the seasons of your emotions pass, for example. Or you might visualise sitting on the shore of a beach as the sea gently crashes forth and drags back, taking your worries with it. Experiment until what you see in your mind's eye resonates for you.

KONFLIKTFÄHIGKEIT

/kɔnflɪk'tˈfɛːɪçkaɪt/ | noun | German
1. literally 'conflictability'; the capacity to overcome disagreements,
find a fair solution and promote tolerance

Our ability to display patience and poise is often most critically tested, not by external circumstances or inconveniences, but by other individuals. Infamous French existentialist, Jean-Paul Sartre, is often quoted for his pithy one-liner that *l'enfer, c'est les autres* or 'hell is other people'. Sartre's idea here was not so much that people are intrinsically hellish, but more that they cause us to recognise uncomfortable things about ourselves – which causes us conflict. Either way, while we depend upon others to survive and desire closeness with them in all kinds of ways, each of us will know that getting along with people is often plagued with strife.

The stoic and sensible German people have a concept that might just offer a solution to this perpetual dance between closeness and recoil: *konfliktfähigkeit* or 'conflictability'. This term captures the idea that, in many ways, conflict between individuals and groups is inevitable, but that this need not mean we blunder through these situations unprepared and bewildered. Instead, as with most things, we can build up certain strategies and capacities for facing conflict with wisdom, tolerance, proficiency and good grace.

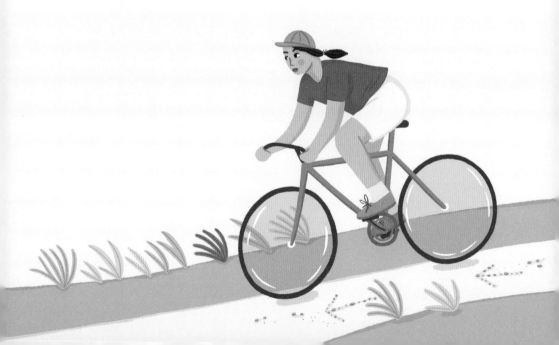

It would be unrealistic of any of us to believe that we will always act in perfect equanimity and live our days in Buddhist-like acceptance of all others, so there is something appealingly pragmatic about *konfliktfähigkeit*. It says that, sure, conflict happens, but that does not mean we cannot get better at it. The trick to *konfliktfähigkeit* is that we recognise and are honest about potential conflicts. In this way we become better able to manage them. *Konfliktfähigkeit* therefore not only helps us to resolve clashes in the moment, but it is also a kind of philosophy that can underpin all our interactions. Inevitable disagreements crop up between people, but this need not stop us exercising a spirit of openness and willing, nor should it prevent us from taking constructive steps forwards together. Rather than becoming avoidant or, worse, passive aggressive, with *konfliktfähigkeit* we can face up to disputes with patience and poise.

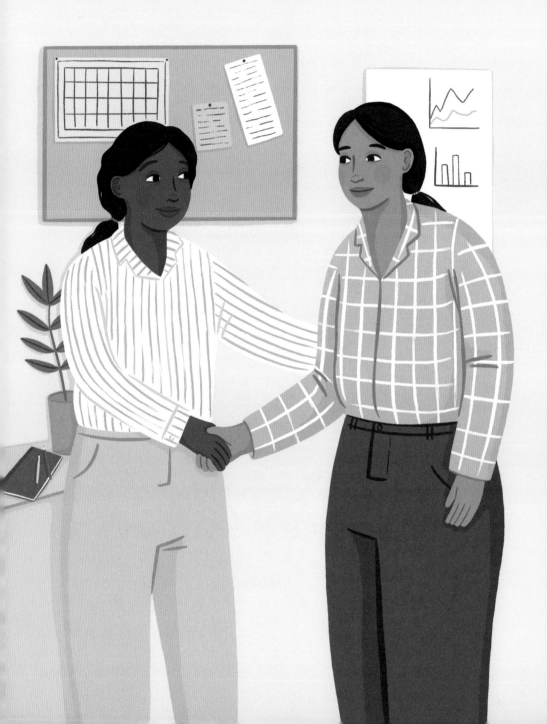

TRY THIS...

Communicate with *Konfliktfähigkeit*

While *konfliktfähigkeit* sounds like a nice idea, it may well prove problematic to put into practise. We are all liable to 'see red' or to become hot headed when we face a disagreement. In these moments, few of us are readily able to speak or act from a place of compassion and good grace.

This is precisely why, when tensions run high, it is important that we have strategies in place and systems of communication that can helpfully scaffold our disagreements and keep things peaceful. One well-known methodology for doing exactly this is the process of *nonviolent communication*, developed by Marshall B Rosenberg. This deeply compassionate mode of communication seeks to avoid hurtful or 'violent' interactions in a diverse range of life domains. It therefore represents what we can think of as an advanced, formalised process of *konfliktfähigkeit*. It involves calm observation of the situation, as well as stating our feelings and needs before making a request of the other person. Easy to say, but may well take a great deal of practise (it is possible to train and gain qualifications in nonviolent communication).

Even if we are not well versed in this specific formal process, however, we can all take simple steps to mindfully approach a difficult conversation with genuine serenity and compassion.

Be sure to pause

An important initial step in any potential conflict situation is to simply pause and reflect in the moment. Are you falling out, or about to fall out with a partner, colleague or relative? Is someone's behaviour grating on you? Taking a moment, even very briefly, to ensure you have made as accurate as possible an assessment of what is taking place. This will give you the best chance of gauging your own actions and reactions.

Be clear about your aims

Do you wish to get the other person to do something, or simply want them to understand your viewpoint? It is vital to be crystal clear about this so as to avoid simply ranting, and also to give the best chance of getting an outcome that is beneficial to all. If you realise you are actually without a specific aim – as in there is nothing to gain on either side from the discussion – then it may be best to walk away altogether.

Be ready to act compassionately

Only once you have paused to calmly assess the situation, and considered what the hoped-for outcome might be, comes the time to act. Take a deep breath and express your aims to the other person, remaining aware that their own aims might be quite different, and that the best you might sometimes hope for is simply to 'agree to disagree'.

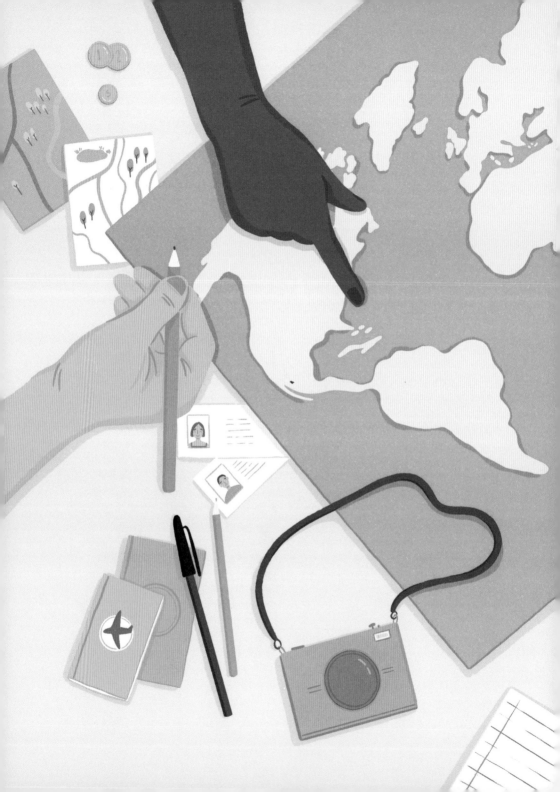

VOORPRET

/ˈvoːr.prɛt/ | noun | Dutch
1. pre-fun; the joy of anticipation

It is often said that patience is a virtue. For the Dutch people, when done right, patience can also make for a ruddy good time. This is because the Dutch understand the pleasure of 'pre-fun' or *voorpret*. (The Germans have a similar noun, *vorfreude* meaning a similar kind of joyful anticipation, derived from imagining a future pleasure).

Most of us can think of at least one exciting thing we have on the horizon to feel good about (and, if not, maybe it is time to get something in the calendar!). Perhaps it is a weekend away, or a more far-flung and exotic trip, a visit from friends or loved ones, or a new creative project you want to start. The idea of *voorpret* is that, rather than lamenting the days, weeks or months we have to wait before said pleasure arrives – we bask in this waiting period.

Taking pleasure in waiting seems a rather odd concept in our high-speed world of instant gratification. In the modern day we rarely have to wait long for anything, be it the latest album from a band we love (we can download it instantly), our next hot meal (it can be bicycled to our door within the hour) or even our next hot date (we can connect with someone in five seconds flat through a dating app). As such, the times when we are forced to wait – such as being kept on hold when we phone the bank, for example – have become more frustrating than ever. Yet finding the pleasure in pre-fun is far more conducive to calm than biting our fingernails with impatience.

Turns out that *voorpret* is not simply a fanciful idea, but is psychologically sound. In response to a range of studies confirming the enjoyment people garner from *recalling* pleasant events, one pair of psychological researchers conducted a range of experiments indicating that the *anticipation* of positive events, such as holidays, may equally impact our overall satisfaction with life. What better reason to put some fun, and some pre-fun, on the agenda?

TRY THIS...

Make Pre-fun Part of your Plans

Once we realise that it is not only the moment of a joyful experience itself that is ours to savour, but also the time that leads up to and follows it (in the spirit of *voorpret*), then we see that life can be likened to a rather ripe orange just waiting to be squeezed of its juicy goodness.

Got a happy event shimmering on your horizon? Lucky you, you have the chance to practise the art of *voorpret* and experience the pleasure of pre-fun. Don't have anything in mind? Plan in both the fun and the pre-fun by making a date in your diary now for a joyful occasion in the future, even if it is something simple like a trip to a gallery or shopping date with a friend.

Three ways to practise the art of voorpret:

1. **Schedule in some fun.** This is a simple yet essential first step to experiencing voorpret. Many of us are guilty of stringently packing our calendars with duties like dental appointments, work meetings, supermarket shops and collecting things

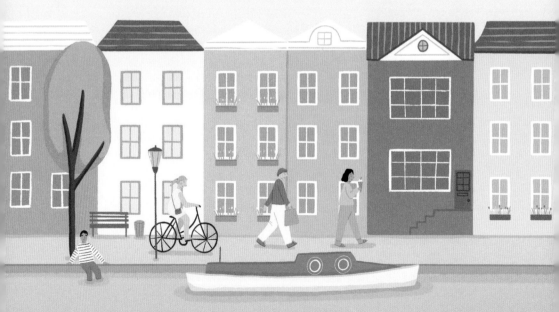

from the dry cleaners. How many of us make time to schedule in simple pleasures? Sure, we might have major birthdays or holidays marked down, but what if we committed to scheduling at least one small fun event per week? That would make for a whole lot more *voorpret*.

2. **Reflective writing.** This is perhaps the number one way that we can refocus on the joys in our life – past, present or future. Start with the prompt: '*I am looking forward to...*' and then describe as many of the exciting specifics of a particular event or occasion as possible, and why you are looking forward to them. You can revisit this writing as many times as you like in the lead up to the event to stimulate your feelings of *voorpret*, and also revisit it after (to recall and relive the excitement).

3. **Set reminders in your calendar.** While we might have the best intentions to stick to points 1 and 2, we all know that life gets in the way and conflicting commitments can stack up. In this moment (while you hopefully have the impetus to create more of a sense of *voorpret* in your life), pop a weekly or monthly alert in your electronic calendar. It might simply say, '*Practise voorpret today!*'. In this way, whatever good thing happens to be on the horizon at that future moment, you will be prompted to anticipate it with pleasure. Easy.

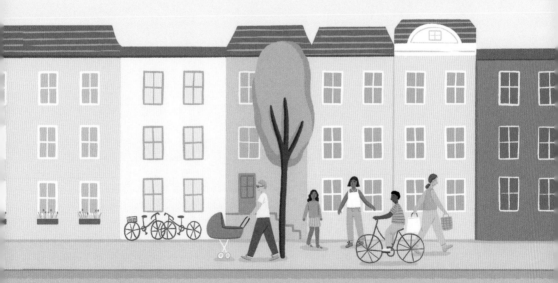

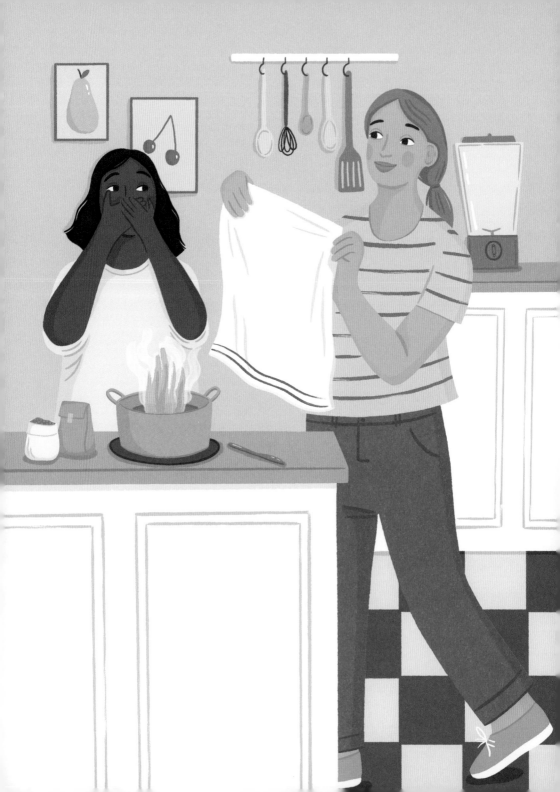

DESENRASCANÇO

/ˌdi.zɐ̃j.ʁɐʃ.ˈkɐ̃.su/ | noun | Portuguese

1. disentanglement
2. the ability to improvise a quick solution

Sometimes our sense of poise is the result of meticulous planning and forward thinking, yet sometimes we must simply react with confidence to the situation at hand – and centre on a swift solution in the moment. For the Portuguese, the noun *desenrascanço* evokes this talent for in-the-moment ingenuity and unflustered resourcefulness when in a bind.

Desenrascanço is, literally, the ability to 'disentangle' oneself from a tricky situation by finding a crafty remedy to the problem. It is a cherished virtue that many believe reflects the national culture of Portugal. In English, the closest translation of this characteristic of clever composure might be the ability to 'muddle through' – but this does not quite capture the highly positive nature of the word.

It is a matter of pride for the Portuguese to exercise the spirit of *desenrascanço*; to devise imaginative solutions when faced with the toughest of conundrums, even when one does not have the correct tools, or even much time. It is the ability to spot a clear answer amid a great big mess – and to stay calm in the process.

This capacity for spur-of-the-moment problem solving is a long-held virtue recognised both by the Portuguese themselves and their neighbours. It is said that, for many centuries, sailing ships across Europe would aim to employ at least one Portuguese crew member, to add this uniquely Portuguese talent for *desenrascanço* to their combined skillset should anything go wrong at sea.

Desenrascanço is a celebration of the ways in which it is possible to face life head on, safe in the knowledge that we have all we need to face even the most puzzling of pitfalls. It is the opposite of getting bogged down by excessive planning, and is rather an attitude of simply getting on with things, trusting that you will find the solution you need, when you need it.

A Map of Calm

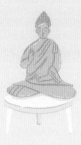

Although our journey through this book has drawn to a close, a bigger journey is just beginning. Across the globe, individuals, communities and scholars are coming together with increasing enthusiasm to share the diverse ways in which we can describe – and experience – life, and live it well.

Dr Tim Lomas is a positive psychologist and founder of *The Happy Words Project*. The project has an 'ambitious and uplifting aim' Dr Lomas says; to gather and create an online resource of 'untranslatable words relating to wellbeing from across the world's languages'. Through research and crowd-sourced suggestions, so far more than 1,000 words have been identified (www.drtimlomas.com/lexicography). This has created a 'detailed conceptual "map" of our experiential world – particularly as it relates to wellbeing'.

'One of the most prominent and important "regions" of this world' Dr Lomas says, 'is that of calmness and serenity, which includes a wealth of precious feelings'. He advocates that, by familarising ourselves with these feelings, 'not only do we gain a greater appreciation and understanding of other cultures (which is of course valuable in itself), but also of our own experiential world'. This can help in 'developing a greater vocabulary with which to represent and conceptualise our lives, allowing us to articulate experiences' that we may have 'previously struggled' to name, or even understand.

Many words and concepts, Dr Lomas says, that may be 'lacking an exact equivalent in our own tongue can help enrich our conceptual understanding of wellbeing, and even our lived experience of it'. 'Even more tantalisingly' he adds, 'by engaging with such words, we may even be led into new dimensions of the world, with language opening up new possibilities for living'.

When we take the time to understand how serenity, calm and wellbeing more broadly manifest around the world (just as we have in this book) we can come to appreciate these experiences in wholly new – and perhaps truly transformative – ways.

Extend the Journey

You can find out a little more about the words and
concepts featured in this book, as well as the research
behind them, with these further resources.

FURTHER READING

Dr Tim Lomas, *The Happiness Dictionary: Words from Around the World to Help Us Lead a Richer Life,* Piatkus, 2018.

Tiffany Watt Smith, *The Book of Human Emotions: An Encyclopedia of Feeling from Anger to Wanderlust,* Wellcome Collection, 2015.

TAKE A DIP... WAYS WE BATHE

Saylee Deshmukh, Mahesh Vyas, Hitesh Vyas, Dwivedi R R, 'Concept of Lifestyle in Ayurveda Classics', *Global Journal of Research on Medicinal Plants & Indigenous Medicine,* vol. 4(2), 2015, 30–37.

Shevchuk, Nikolai A, 'Adapted cold shower as a potential treatment for depression.' *Medical Hypotheses* 70, no. 5, 2008, 995–1001.

THE SERENITY OF SLUMBER

'The Benefits of Slumber: Why You Need a Good Night's Sleep', *News in Health,* National Institutes of Health, 2013, https://newsinhealth.nih.gov/2013/04/benefits-slumber

SHU

Joseph Emmanuel D. Sta. Maria, 'Shu and Zhong as the Virtue of the Golden Rule: A Confucian Contribution to Contemporary Virtue Ethics', *Asian Philosophy* 27, no. 2, 2017, 100–111.

Cendri A. Hutcherson, Emma M. Seppala, and James J. Gross, 'Loving-Kindness Meditation Increases Social Connectedness.', *Emotion 8,* no. 5, 2008, 720–24.

SATI

Tamara Ditrich, 'Situating the Concept of Mindfulness in the Theravāda Tradition', *Asian Studies 4,* no. 2, 2016, 15.

AYLIAK

'Plovdiv Together 2019', Municipal Foundation Plovdiv 2019, http://www.ecoc2019bulgaria.eu/images/content/33/app_en_plovdiv.pdf

FLOW

Mihaly Csikszentmihalyi and Jeanne Nakamura, 'Effortless attention in everyday life: A systematic phenomenology', *Effortless Attention: A New Perspective in the Cognitive Science of Attention and Action,* ed. Bryan Bruya, MIT Press, 2010.

Mihaly Csikszentmihalyi, *Flow: The Classic Work on How to Achieve Happiness,* London: Rider, 2002.

HO'OPONOPONO

Dennis P. Nishihare, 'Culture, Counseling and Ho'oponopono: An Ancient Model in a Modern Context', *Personnel and Guidance Journal,* vol. 56, issue 9, 1978, pp. 562–566.

APRAMĀDA

Dr Tim Lomas, *Translating Happiness: A Cross-Cultural Lexicon of Well-Being,* MIT Press, 2018, p.103.
The Triratna Dharma Training Course for Mitras – Year Four, 2012, Triratna Buddhist Community, pp. 172–177, http://www.thebuddhistcentre.com.

CAPOEIRA

John J. Crocitti , and Monique Vallance, *Brazil Today: An Encyclopedia of Life in the Republic,* ABC-CLIO, 2012, pp. 130–132.

The Organisation for Economic Co-operation and Development (OECD), 'Better Life Index', http://www.oecdbetterlifeindex.org/countries/brazil/

Soul Capoeira blog, 2008, http://www.soulcapoeira.org/blog/bruxas-blog/warming-up-and-stretching-in-capoeira/

PRĀNĀYĀMA

Maheshkumar Kuppusamy et al., 'Effects of Bhramari Pranayama on Health – A Systematic Review', *Journal of Traditional and Complementary Medicine* 8, no. 1, 2018, 11–16.

HÓZHÓ

Michelle Kahn-John and Mary Koithan. 'Living in health, harmony, and beauty: The Diné (Navajo) Hózhó wellness philosophy.' *Global Advances in Health and Medicine 4,* no. 3, 2015, 24–30.

HASYA YOGA
Sandra Manninen et al., 'Social Laughter Triggers
Endogenous Opioid Release in Humans', *Journal of
Neuroscience* 37, no. 25, 21 June 2017, 6125-31.
Laughter Yoga International,
https://laughteryoga.org/laughter-yoga/
about-laughter-yoga/

FIKA
Lynda Balslev, *The Little Book of Fika: The Uplifting
Daily Ritual of the Swedish Coffee Break,*
Andrews McMeel Publishing, 2018.

MITZVAH
Tzvi Freeman, 'What is a Mitzvah: The State of Being
Connected', Chabad.org,
https://www.chabad.org/library/article_cdo/aid/1438516/
jewish/Mitzvah.htm

Lynn E. Alden and Jennifer L. Trew, 'If It Makes
You Happy: Engaging in Kind Acts Increases
Positive Affect in Socially Anxious Individuals',
Emotion 13, no. 1, February 2013, 64-75.

UTEPILS
An Enthusiastic's Lexicon blog, 2001,
https://enthusiastslexicon.wordpress.
com/2011/03/08/utepils/

SADHANA
Alan Verdegraal, 'Sadhana' in *Tantra: The Magazine,*
1994, Issue #8, pp. 22-23.

NUCHI GUSUI
**Donald Craig Willcox, Giovanni Scapagnini, and
Bradley J. Willcox,** 'Healthy Aging Diets Other than
the Mediterranean: A Focus on the Okinawan Diet',
Mechanisms of Ageing and Development,
Mediterranean Diet and Inflammaging in the elderly,
136-137, 1 March 2014, 148-62.

FREDAGSMYS
Catherine Edwards, 'Swedish word of the day',
The Local SE,
https://www.thelocal.se/20190208/swedish-word-of-
the-day-fredagsmys

FJAKA
Kristin Vuković, 'Dalmatia's Fjaka State of Mind,
BBC.com,
http://www.bbc.com/travel/story/20180118-dalmatias-
fjaka-state-of-mind

MORGENFRISK
P. Tysoe, 'The effect on staff of essential oil
burners in extended care settings',
International Journal of Nursing Practice,
vol. 6, no. 2, 2000, pp. 110-112.

GAMAN
Mira Shimabukuro, '"Me Inwardly, Before I Dared":
Japanese Americans Writing-to-Gaman',
College English 73, no. 6, 2011, 648-71.

BELUM
Josafina Lara Chavez, 'Belum', Stories from Indonesia,
Peace Corps website,
https://www.peacecorps.gov/indonesia/stories/belum/

UPEKṢĀ
Bhikkhu Bodhi, 'Toward a Threshold of Understanding',
Access to Insight (BCBS Edition), 5 June 2010,
http://www.accesstoinsight.org/lib/authors/bodhi/
bps-essay_30.html

KONFLIKTFÄHIGKEIT
Marshall B. Rosenberg, *Nonviolent Communication:
A language of life,* Encinitas, CA: Puddle
Dancer Press, 2015.

VOORPRET
Leaf Van Boven and Laurence Ashworth,
'Looking Forward, Looking Back: Anticipation
Is More Evocative than Retrospection.',
Journal of Experimental Psychology:
General 136, no. 2, 2007, 289-300.

DESENRASCANÇO
*Portugal Society & Culture Complete Report:
An All-Inclusive Profile Combining All of
Our Society and Culture Reports,*
World Trade Press, 2010, p.17.

About the Author

Megan C Hayes is an author and academic and has spent a decade studying and researching writing and the psychology of happiness. Megan's interdisciplinary PhD explored writing as a tool to promote and support psychological wellbeing, and she has shared her research in the UK, USA, and Europe, including papers in The International Journal of Wellbeing and Writing in Practice: The Journal of Creative Writing Research. From this research Megan pioneered the Positive Journal® approach to personal writing (www.positivejournal.org)—a way to put wellbeing into words. She is a happy wayfarer who calls the globe home, but wherever she is she can usually be found drinking tea and reading five books at once.

About the Illustrator

Amelia Flower is a British illustrator, who works with clients worldwide in creating captivating and effective illustrations. Amelia's illustration work often takes inspiration from people-watching, and observing social situations and characters, starting many illustrations by sketching from life to capture the spirt of a scene or character. Amelia has illustrated several books.

Thanks

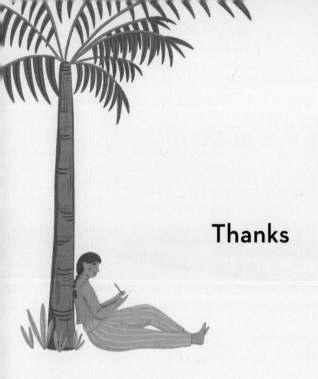

This book has been a truly collaborative affair and I am indebted
to so many for their help in bringing it together.

Thanks to Philippa Wilkinson, Julia Shone, the wider team at
White Lion Publishing/The Quarto Group and to my agent
Jane Graham Maw for your efforts at every stage of the project.

Thanks once again to Lauren Gurteen for your invaluable help in
crafting the pronunciations of these words. Special thanks to Sanna
Bertilsson for sharing your family recipe for Swedish cinnamon buns,
showing me how to make them and – of course – for introducing me
to the joys of *fredagsmys*. Thanks also to Tim Lomas for generously
allowing me to feature your research here, for your kindness and
for your excellent work in this area.

As always, I am grateful to my family and friends for discussing
ideas with me, providing inspiration and bolstering me time
and again (in writing and in life).

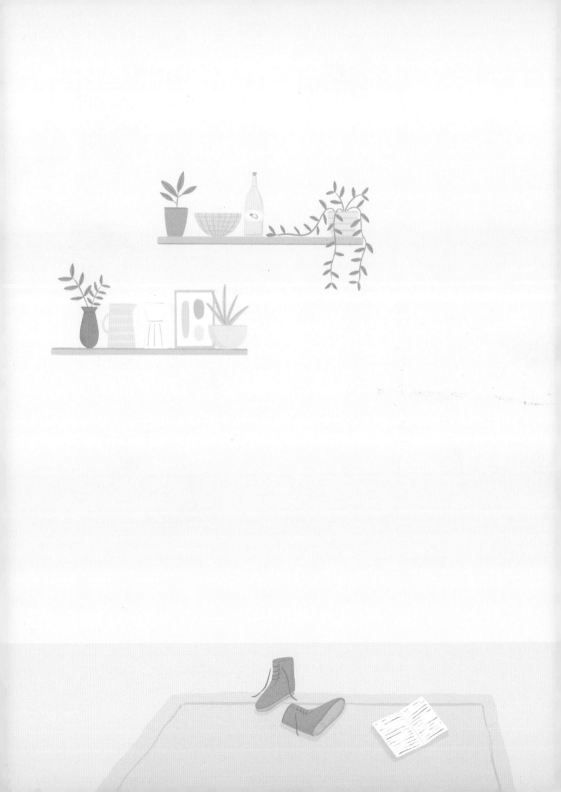